Workbook for

Providing Home Care

A Textbook for Home Health Aides

THIRD EDITION

By Hartman Publishing, Inc.

Credits

MANAGING EDITOR
Susan Alvare

COVER DESIGNER
Kirsten Browne

INTERIOR DESIGNER
Thaddeus Castillo

ILLUSTRATOR
Thaddeus Castillo

COMPOSITION
Thaddeus Castillo

PROOFREADERS
Andrea Bithell
Michele Wiedemer

Notice to Readers

Though the guidelines and procedures contained in this text are based on consultations with healthcare profession-als, they should not be considered absolute recommendations. The instructor and readers should follow employer, local, state, and federal guidelines concerning healthcare practices. These guidelines change, and it is the reader's responsibility to be aware of these changes and of the policies and procedures of her or his healthcare facility.

The publisher, author, editors, and reviewers cannot accept any responsibility for errors or omissions or for any con-sequences from application of the information in this book and make no warranty, expressed or implied, with respect to the contents of the book. The publisher does not warrant or guarantee any of the products described here-in or perform any analysis in connection with any of the product information contained herein.

Copyright Information

Table of Contents

Preface

Welcome to the *Workbook for Providing Home Care: A Textbook for Home Health Aides*! This workbook is designed to help you review what you have learned from reading your textbook. For this reason, the workbook is organized around learning objectives, just like the textbook and even your instructor's teaching material.

These learning objectives work as a built-in study guide. After completing the exercises for each learning objective in the workbook, ask yourself if you can DO what that learning objective describes.

If you can, move on to the next learning objective. If you cannot, just go back to the textbook, reread that learning objective, and try again.

We have provided procedure checklists close to the end of the workbook. The answers to the workbook exercises are in your instructor's teaching guide.

Happy Learning!

1

Home Care and the Healthcare System

1. Describe the structure of the healthcare system and describe ways it is changing

Matching.

For each of the following terms, write the letter of the correct definition from the list below.

1. _____ HMOs (health maintenance organizations)

2. _____ Facilities

3. _____ Managed care

4. _____ Payers

5. _____ PPOs (preferred provider organizations)

6. _____ Providers

7. _____ Traditional insurance companies

a. Cost control strategies that are replacing traditional insurance companies

b. People or organizations that provide health care

c. Places where care is delivered or administered

d. A health plan which states that clients must use a particular doctor or group of doctors

e. People or organizations paying for healthcare services

f. A network of providers that contract to provide health services to a group of people

g. Companies that offer plans that pay for health care for plan members

Multiple Choice.

Circle the letter of the answer that best completes the statement or answers the question.

8. Another name for a long-term care (LTC) facility is:
   a. Nursing home
   b. Home health care
   c. Assisted living facility
   d. Adult daycare facility

9. Assisted living facilities are initially for:
   a. Clients who need around-the-clock intensive care
   b. Clients who need some help with daily care
   c. Clients who will die within six months
   d. Clients who need to be in an acute care facility

10. Care given by a specialist to restore or improve function after an illness or injury is called:
    a. Acute care
    b. Subacute care
    c. Rehabilitation
    d. Hospice care

11. Care given to people who have six months or less to live is called:
    a. Acute care
    b. Subacute care
    c. Rehabilitation
    d. Hospice care

2. Explain Medicare and Medicaid, and list when Medicare recipients may receive home care

True or False.

Mark each statement with either a "T" for true or an "F" for false.

1. _____ To qualify for home health care, Medicare recipients must be unable to leave home.

2. _____ Medicare will pay for any care that the recipient desires.

3. _____ Medicare will only cover people aged 65 or older.

4. _____ Medicaid is a medical assistance pro-gram for low-income people.

5. _____ Home health care is never covered by Medicare.

6. _____ Medicare has two parts: hospital insurance and medical insurance.

7. _____ Medicare pays for 100% of all home care.

3. Explain the purpose of and need for home health care

Fill in the Blank.

1. Home care is less

   _____

   than a long hospital or nursing home stay.

2. The growing numbers of

   _____ and

   _____

   people are also creating a demand for home care services.

3. Home services will be needed to provide continued care and assistance as chronic ill-nesses progress. For example,

   _____ is a

   chronic illness that is infecting more and more people and may require in-home assistance.

4. One of the most important reasons for health care in the home is that most people who are ill or disabled feel more comfortable at _____.

4. List key events in the history of home care services

Multiple Choice.

1. What event happened in 1959 to note the need for home health care?

   a. Homemakers were ordered to war and were therefore unable to help out at home.

   b. A national conference on homemaker services was held.

   c. The Medicare program was created.

   d. A national holiday commemorating homemakers was established.

2. When was Medicare created?

   a. 1912

   b. 1996

   c. 1965

   d. 1959

3. Why has interest in home health care increased in recent years?

   a. The population of elderly people and people with chronic diseases grew.

   b. Many hospitals closed due to lack of business.

   c. Healthcare costs decreased dramatically.

   d. Insurance companies often cover 100% of the costs of home health care.

4. What is the function of a DRG (diagnostic related group)?

   a. It pairs people with like illnesses togeth-er to form a support system.

   b. It offers formal training for people with disabilities to reenter the workplace.

   c. It specifies the treatment cost that Medicare or Medicaid will pay for vari-ous diagnoses.

   d. It obtains financial assistance for people with debilitating illnesses.

5. Identify the basic methods of payment for home health services

Short Answer.

Identify three of the five basic methods of payment for home health services and write a short description of each.

_____

_____

_____

_____

_____

_____

_____

_____

_____

_____

_____

_____

_____

_____

_____

_____

_____

_____

_____

6. Describe a typical home health agency

Labeling.

Fill in the four blanks below to complete the diagram of a typical home health agency. Some blanks have already been filled in for you.

7. Explain how working for a home health agency is different from working in other types of facilities

Fill in the Blank.

1. Be aware of personal

_____

when you are traveling alone to visit clients.

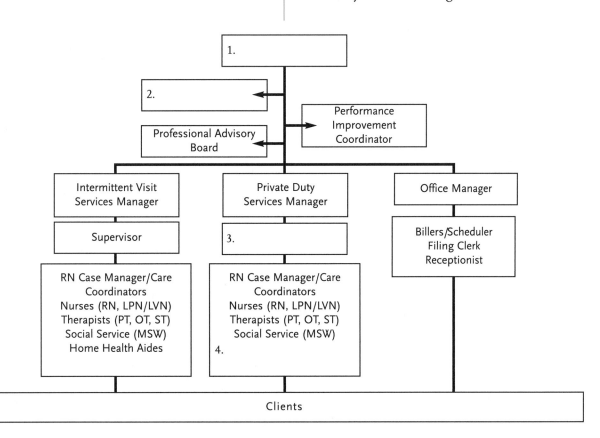

2. You may have a lot more contact with clients' _____ in the home than you would in a facility.

3. Your supervisor will monitor your work, but you will spend most of your hours working with clients without direct supervision. Thus, you must be

    _____.

4. Good written and verbal

    _____

    skills are important.

5. You will need to be

    _____

    in order to adapt to the changes in environment.

6. In a client's home, you are a

    _____.

    Be respectful of the client's property and customs.

2

The Home Health Aide and Care Team

1. Identify the role of each healthcare team member

Matching.

1. _____ Case Manager or Supervisor
2. _____ Home Health Aide (HHA)
3. _____ Medical Social Worker (MSW)
4. _____ Occupational Therapist (OT)
5. _____ Physical Therapist (PT)
6. _____ Physician or Doctor (MD)
7. _____ Registered Dietitian (RDT) or Nutritionist
8. _____ Registered Nurse (RN)
9. _____ Speech Language Pathologist (SLP) or Speech Therapist
10. _____ Client

a. Administers therapy in an effort to improve the client's physical status

b. Coordinates, manages, and provides care, as well as supervising HHAs and developing the HHA assignments

c. Diagnoses disease or disability and prescribes treatment

d. Formulates and supervises each client's care plan and makes changes to the care plan when necessary

e. Helps clients get support services, such as counseling

f. Performs delegated tasks, such as taking vital signs, providing personal care, and reporting observations to other care team members

g. Teaches clients and their families about diets to improve health and manage illness

h. Teaches exercises to help the client improve or overcome speech impediments

i. The care team revolves around this person and his or her condition, treatment, and progress.

j. Trains clients to compensate for disabilities during ADLs and other activities

2. Define the client care plan and explain its purpose

True or False.

1. _____ The purpose of the client care plan is to give suggestions for care, which the home health aide can customize for each client.

2. _____ Activities that are not listed on the care plan should not be performed without permission from the supervisor.

3. Describe how each team member contributes to the care plan

Short Answer.

List contributions that each of the following team members might make in developing the care plan.

1. Home Health Aide (HHA)

   _____

   _____

   _____

2. Case Manager or Supervisor

   _____

   _____

   _____

3. Physician (MD)

_____

_____

_____

_____

4. Medical Social Worker (MSW)

_____

_____

_____

_____

4. Describe the role of the home health aide and explain typical tasks performed

Short Answer.

List and give examples of two ways in which home health aides provide services to their clients.

_____

_____

_____

_____

_____

_____

_____

5. Identify tasks outside the scope of practice for home health aides

True or False.

1. _____ Home health aides never administer medications unless they are trained and assigned to do so.

2. _____ Home health aides are trained to perform "invasive" procedures.

3. _____ Home health aides should ignore any requests that are outside of their scope of practice.

4. _____ Home health aides must not accept any request that is not part of their job description or that is not on the assignment sheet.

5. _____ The correct way to deal with unacceptable requests is to explain why the request cannot be met, and report it to the supervisor.

6. _____ Home health aides should not perform procedures that require sterile technique.

7. _____ It is acceptable for home health aides to prescribe certain medications, if they have permission from their supervisor.

8. _____ Home health aides should only inform the client or family of the diagnosis or medical treatment plan if the client asks.

9. _____ Home health aides may perform any task for which they have been trained, even if it is not part of their assignment.

6. List the federal regulations that apply to home health aides

Fill in the Blank.

1. Home health aides must complete

_____

hours of training and/or pass a

_____

before they begin working.

2. Home health aides must have at least 12 hours of

_____

every year.

3. It is the responsibility of the

_____ to

successfully complete the required in-service training each year.

4. _____ is the federal government agency that makes rules to protect workers from hazards on the job.

7. Describe the purpose of the chain of command

Labeling.

Fill in the blanks to complete the diagram of the chain of command.

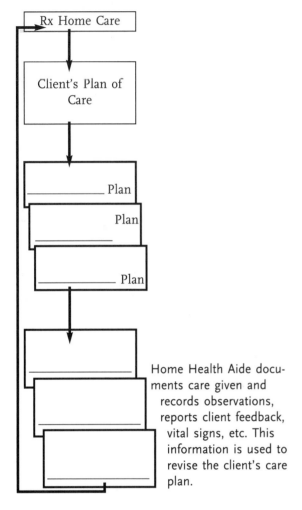

Short Answer

Using the above diagram, answer the following questions.

1. Who orders home care for a client?

_____

_____

2. Who coordinates the plan of care?

_____

_____

3. Who are three care team members who might receive assignments?

_____

_____

_____

4. What are three types of documentation used for feedback in care planning?

_____

_____

_____

8. Define policies and procedures and explain why they are important

Short Answer.

List five examples of common policies and procedures at home health agencies.

1. _____

2. _____

3. _____

4. _____

5. _____

9. List examples of a professional relationship with a client and an employer

Short Answer.

Read each of the following scenarios and answer the questions.

1. Kathy, a home health aide, wakes up late and decides to skip her morning shower to make up for lost time. She also skips breakfast because she wants to make her first assignment on time. Because she is feeling so rushed, she forgets to respond when her client says, "Good morning." Instead, she complains to her client about her sleepless night, headache, and lack of breakfast.

   Is Kathy behaving in a professional manner?

   _____

   _____

What should she have done instead?

_____

_____

_____

_____

2. At her next client's home, Kathy asks to use the restroom. She washes her hands carefully when she is finished, and begins to prepare her client's lunch. She listens to her client talk about his grandchildren's visit the day before, and encourages her client to share photographs of the grandchildren. As Kathy is leaving, her client offers her a gift. Kathy politely refuses the gift and explains that it is against her agency's policy.

List all the examples of Kathy's professional behavior.

_____

_____

_____

_____

_____

_____

3. Steve, a home health aide, runs out of time at one client's home and is unable to finish his assignment. When his supervisor finds out, she tells him that he needs to work more efficiently. This makes Steve very upset, and he begins to wonder if his job is worth all the criticism he seems to be getting.

Is Steve behaving in professionally?

_____

What should he have done instead?

_____

_____

_____

_____

4. At his next meeting with his supervisor, Steve explains why he was unable to finish his assignment and asks his supervisor for suggestions. She shows him how to organize his time more efficiently. After asking several more questions, Steve feels that he now understands how to work more effectively. Being able to communicate in a positive way with his supervisor improves Steve's attitude about his job.

List all the examples of Steve's professional behavior.

_____

_____

_____

_____

_____

_____

_____

10. Demonstrate how to organize care assignments

Short Answer.

1. Discuss why it is important to organize your work.

_____

_____

_____

_____

_____

_____

_____

2. Why should you include the client in planning your schedule?

_____

_____

_____

_____

_____

_____

11. Demonstrate good personal grooming habits

Word Search.

Complete each of the following sentences and then find the answers in the word search.

1. Good _____
makes you feel great and others feel good
about you.

2. _____ or
_____
daily are important parts of good grooming.

3. Wash and iron your
_____
regularly.

4. Do not wear clothes that are too
_____ .

5. Long
_____
should be tied back in a bun or ponytail.

6. Use _____
or anti-perspirant every day.

7. Do not wear
_____ as
some clients may not be tolerant of some
odors.

8. Never wear
_____ that
is too large or gets in the way.

9. No _____
should be visible.

10. Keep fingernails short and
_____ .

11. Do not wear artificial
_____ .

12. Wear little or no
_____ .

h	j	e	w	e	l	r	y	b	w	t	y	s
p	u	e	k	a	m	m	s	y	n	g	l	x
o	i	e	o	z	y	l	d	a	g	e	r	g
z	e	h	m	p	i	n	r	a	t	h	a	h
s	m	k	z	a	f	o	b	p	r	j	t	g
e	u	h	n	e	d	w	i	c	l	e	a	n
h	f	s	b	o	e	e	d	g	u	r	t	i
t	r	m	e	x	k	u	x	t	d	b	t	r
o	e	d	r	e	t	l	o	s	o	v	o	e
l	p	i	w	u	m	x	t	y	r	t	o	w
c	a	b	a	t	h	i	n	g	y	j	s	o
h	e	j	r	g	n	i	m	o	o	r	g	h
r	o	l	k	h	w	c	s	u	l	j	y	s

12. Identify personal qualities a home health aide must have

Short Answer.

From this learning objective in the textbook, pick three qualities that you believe you can improve in yourself, and describe how you will improve on these qualities.

1. _____
_____
_____

2. _____
_____
_____

3. _____
_____
_____

13. Identify an employer's responsibilities

Short Answer.

List and describe four responsibilities of the employer to the home health aide.

1. _____
_____

2. _____
_____

3. _____
_____

4. _____
_____

3

Legal and Ethical Issues

1. Define the terms "ethics" and "laws" and list examples of legal and ethical behavior

Short Answer.

Read each of the following scenarios and answer the questions.

1. Sarah, a home health aide, is out shopping with her friends. One of them asks her if she likes her job, and she responds enthusiastically. She proceeds to relate to them that her client, Mrs. Daly, has Alzheimer's disease and has to be reminded of her name several times a day, as she is apt to forget it.

   Did Sarah behave in a legal and ethical manner? Why or why not?

   _____

   _____

   _____

   _____

   _____

2. Caroyl, a home health aide, finishes her duties for the day early. Her client, Mr. Leach, tells her how pleased he is with her work. He says that she is the first aide that has made him feel so comfortable and well taken care of. He gives her a little box of candy and says it is for all the hard work she has done. Caroyl initially refuses, but after he insists, she takes it from him, thanking him.

   Did Caroyl behave in a legal and ethical manner? Why or why not?

   _____

   _____

   _____

   _____

   _____

3. Mark, a home health aide, has been working for Mrs. Hedman for almost a year. Her family is visiting from out-of-state and Mark meets her daughter, Susan, for the first time. During the course of conversation, Susan asks Mark to come have a drink with her so that they can talk about her mother's case in a more relaxed environment. Mark tells her that he can go out for a short while. They arrange to meet.

   Did Mark behave in a legal and ethical manner? Why or why not?

   _____

   _____

   _____

   _____

   _____

   _____

2. Explain clients' rights and discuss why they are important

True or False.

1. _____ It is okay to abuse a client psychologically, but never verbally or physically.

2. _____ If a home health aide suspects that a client is being abused, he should keep quiet, in order to not get anyone angry at him.

3. _____ Clients have the right to participate in their care planning.

Name: _____

4. _____ Clients should only be informed of obstacles or barriers to their care if they are life-threatening.

5. _____ Neglect is the failure of a caregiver to take proper care of a person.

6. _____ Clients should never know what the agency expects to happen as a result of their care.

Matching.

7. _____ Abuse

8. _____ Active neglect

9. _____ Assault

10. _____ Battery

11. _____ Domestic violence

12. _____ Financial abuse

13. _____ Involuntary seclusion

14. _____ Negligence

15. _____ Passive neglect

16. _____ Physical abuse

17. _____ Psychological abuse

18. _____ Sexual abuse

19. _____ Sexual harassment

20. _____ Substance abuse

21. _____ Verbal abuse

22. _____ Workplace violence

a. Actions or failure to act or provide proper care resulting in injury to a person

b. The use of legal or illegal drugs, cigarettes, or alcohol in a way that harms oneself or others

c. Any unwelcome sexual advance or behavior that creates an intimidating or hostile work environment

d. Purposely harming a person physically, mentally, or emotionally by failing to give needed or correct care

e. Confinement or separation from others without consent

f. Abuse of caregivers or team members by clients or other team members

g. Touching a person without his or her permission

h. Threatening to touch a person without his or her permission

i. Stealing, taking advantage of, or improperly using the money or other assets of another

j. Forcing a person to perform or participate in sexual acts

k. Oral or written words, pictures, or gestures that threaten, embarrass, or insult another person.

l. Any behavior that causes the client to feel threatened, fearful, intimidated, or humiliated

m. Abuse by spouses, intimate partners, or family members

n. Purposely causing physical, mental, or emotional pain or injury to someone

o. Intentional or unintentional treatment that causes harm to a person's body

p. Unintentionally harming a person physically, mentally, or emotionally by failing to give needed or correct care

3. List ways to recognize and report elder abuse and neglect

Short Answer.

1. Name five "suspicious" injuries that should be reported.

_____

_____

_____

_____

_____

2. What are seven signs that could indicate abuse?

_____

_____

_____

_____

_____

3. What are seven signs that could indicate neglect?

_____

_____

_____

_____

_____

_____

4. List examples of behavior supporting and promoting clients' rights

Multiple Choice.

1. When performing a procedure on clients, you should:
   a. Try to distract them so they will not know what you are doing
   b. Explain the procedure fully before performing it
   c. Wait until they are sleeping before you start the procedure
   d. Always notify the physician first

2. If a client refuses to take a bath, you should:
   a. Offer them a prize if they will take the bath
   b. Respect their wishes, but report it to your supervisor
   c. Tell them you are going to leave if they do not comply
   d. Force them to take the bath

3. If another home health aide asks you about your client's care plan, you should:
   a. Explain that you cannot talk or gossip about your client
   b. Tell them about the care plan
   c. Say "I'll tell if you go first."
   d. Tell them only about your client's diet/nutrition plan but nothing else

4. If you suspect your client is being abused, you should:
   a. Open his mail and look through his belongings to find any clues
   b. Call your closest friends and ask their advice
   c. Report it to your supervisor immediately
   d. Check with his relatives first

5. Explain HIPAA and list ways to protect clients' confidentiality

Short Answer.

1. What can happen to healthcare facilities and their employees if they do not follow HIPAA?

_____

_____

_____

_____

_____

_____

2. What can you say to a person who is not part of the care team when they ask you about your client?

_____

_____

_____

_____

_____

_____

6. Discuss and give examples of advance directives

Matching.

1. _____ Advance directives

2. _____ Living will

3. _____ Durable power of attorney for health care

4. _____ Do-not-resuscitate (DNR) order

a. A signed, dated, and witnessed paper that appoints someone else to make the medical decisions for a person in the event he or she becomes unable to do so.

b. States the medical care a person wants, or does not want, in case he or she becomes unable to make those decisions him- or herself.

c. Legal documents that allow people to choose what medical care they wish to have if they cannot make those decisions themselves.

d. A legal document that tells medical professionals not to perform CPR (cardiopulmonary resuscitation).

7. Identify community resources available to help the elderly

Short Answer.

1. What are two ways an HHA can locate community resources for the elderly?

_____

_____

_____

_____

2. Name two people to whom an HHA could refer clients or families.

_____

_____

_____

_____

4

Communication and Cultural Diversity

1. Define communication

Short Answer.

1. List the three basic steps of communication.

_____
_____
_____
_____
_____
_____
_____

2. Why is feedback an important part of communication?

_____
_____
_____
_____
_____
_____
_____

3. With whom must home health aides be able to communicate?

_____
_____
_____
_____
_____

_____
_____
_____

2. Explain verbal and nonverbal communication

Multiple Choice.

1. Which of the following is an example of nonverbal communication?
   a. Asking for a glass of water
   b. Pointing to a glass of water

2. Types of verbal communication include:
   a. Facial expressions
   b. Nodding your head
   c. Speaking
   d. Shrugging your shoulders

3. Types of nonverbal communication include:
   a. Speaking
   b. Facial expressions
   c. Oral reports
   d. Writing

4. Which of the following is an example of a confusing or conflicting message (saying one thing and meaning another)?
   a. Mr. Carter smiles happily and tells you he is excited because his daughter is coming to visit.
   b. Mrs. Sanchez looks like she is in pain. When you ask her about it, she tells you that her back has been bothering her.
   c. Ms. Jones agrees with you when you say it is a nice day, but she looks angry.
   d. Mr. Lee will not watch his favorite TV show. He says he is a little depressed.

Name: _____

5. In the previous question, how would you clarify the confusing or conflicting message?

   a. State what you have observed and ask if the observation is correct.

   b. Ignore the conflicting message and accept what the person has told you.

   c. Ask the person to repeat what he or she has just said.

   d. Tell the person that you know they are not telling the truth.

3. Identify barriers to communication

Crossword.

Across

2. Your client or the family may not understand _____ terminology.

4. Avoid using _____ words that are unprofessional.

6. Be _____ with a client who is difficult to understand.

8. Do not give medical _____ to the client or family.

10. Keep in mind that _____ language is also part of your message, and be aware of it.

11. Make sure you speak clearly, especially if your client is hard of _____.

Down

1. Ask _____ questions to get more information from the client.

3. "Yes" or "no" answers bring the _____ to an end.

5. _____ are phrases that do not really mean anything.

7. Do not offer your personal _____ to the client or family.

9. Avoid asking _____ when your client makes a statement.

4. List ways to make communication accurate and complete

Short Answer.

List six techniques that can help you send and receive clear, complete messages:

1. _____

2. _____

3. _____

4. _____

5. _____

6. _____

5. Describe the difference between facts and opinions

Fact or Opinion.

For each statement, decide whether it is an example of a fact or an opinion. Write "F" for fact or "O" for opinion in the space provided.

1. _____ It is better to take your bath before you eat.

2. _____ You will get depressed if you stay in your pajamas all day.

3. _____ It is not fair for you to give me a present.

4. _____ My agency says I cannot accept a gift.

5. _____ Your care plan calls for snacks between meals.

6. _____ Mr. Ford drinks more coffee than is good for him.

7. _____ Mr. Ford drinks three cups of coffee every morning.

8. _____ Mrs. Myers needs assistance to stand up.

9. _____ Mrs. Myers looks like she is in a lot of pain.

6. Explain how to develop effective interpersonal relationships

True or False.

For each of the following statements, write "T" if the suggestion will help develop good relationships with clients, and write "F" if it will not.

1. _____ Put yourself in other people's shoes.

2. _____ If a subject makes you feel uncomfortable, change the subject.

3. _____ Lean forward in your chair when listening to someone.

4. _____ Do not talk down to your client.

5. _____ Ignore requests that you cannot honor.

6. _____ Tell clients that you know how they feel.

7. _____ Approach the person who is talking.

7. Describe basic medical terminology and approved abbreviations

Matching.

For each of the following abbreviations, write the letter of the correct term from the list below.

1. _____ ac

2. _____ amb

3. _____ B.M.

4. _____ C

5. _____ c/o

6. _____ CPR

7. _____ F

8. _____ ft

9. _____ GI

10. _____ hs

11. _____ I&O

12. _____ NPO

13. _____ OOB

14. _____ pc

15. _____ PRN

16. _____ R

17. _____ ROM

18. _____ SOB

19. _____ VS

20. _____ w/c

a. Fahrenheit degree

b. hours sleep

c. after meals

d. nothing by mouth

e. bowel movement

f. cardiopulmonary resuscitation

g. complains of

h.   range of motion

i.   respirations

j.   vital signs

k.   shortness of breath

l.   before meals

m.   foot

n.   wheelchair

o.   as necessary

p.   intake and output

q.   Celsius degree

r.   out of bed

s.   gastrointestinal

t.   ambulate

8. Explain how to give and receive an accurate oral report of a client's status

True or False.

1. _____ Oral reports are used to report something immediately to the supervisor.

2. _____ Oral reports are never used to discuss the home health aide's observations of the client.

3. _____ Oral reports are only opinions.

4. _____ Before giving an oral report, make notes to help you remember the basic information.

5. _____ It is not necessary to document an oral report.

6. _____ Do not take notes during a supervisor's oral report, since this can be a distraction.

7. _____ Restate what you have been told to make sure you understand it.

8. _____ After giving an oral report, you must make a written report later.

9. _____ Report anything that endangers the client at the next staff meeting.

10. _____ You may use oral reports from other home health aides to help you with a new client.

9. Demonstrate how to report and document factual observations in written or oral form

Labeling.

Looking at the diagram, list examples of observations using each sense.

Smell: _____
_____
_____
_____

Sight: _____
_____
_____
_____

Hearing: _____
_____
_____

Touch: _____
_____
_____
_____

For each of the following, decide whether it is an objective observation (you can see, hear, smell, or touch it) or subjective observation (the client must tell you about it). Write "O" for objective and "S" for subjective.

1. _____ Skin rash

2. _____ Crying

3. _____ Rapid pulse

4. _____ Headache

5. _____ Nausea

6. _____ Vomiting

7. _____ Swelling

8. _____ Cloudy urine

10. Explain why documentation is important and describe how to document visit records and incident reports

Short Answer.

List three reasons why it is essential that you maintain current documentation for your clients.

1. _____
   _____
   _____
   _____
   _____

2. _____
   _____
   _____
   _____
   _____

3. _____
   _____
   _____
   _____
   _____

True or False.

1. _____ A medical chart is a legal document.

2. _____ Medical charts are not proof that care was given to a client.

3. _____ The information in a medical chart is always confidential.

4. _____ Failing to document visits and activities will not cause any harm to the client.

5. _____ If you did not document it, legally you did not do it.

6. _____ Visit notes should be written at the end of the day when there is more time to write.

7. _____ The purpose of visit notes is to serve as a record of the home health aide's visit and the care provided.

8. _____ To help you present your thoughts as briefly and clearly as possible, you should simply write and not spend a lot of time initially thinking about what you are going to write.

9. _____ Include your own thoughts and opinions about the visit in the visit notes.

10. _____ If you make a mistake, erase the mistake or use correction fluid.

11. _____ After completing each day's visit notes, sign your full name, your title, and the date.

12. _____ Incidents must be reported before leaving the client's home.

13. _____ Do not report an incident that makes you feel uncomfortable unless you think it might be a direct threat to you.

14. _____ If your client breaks something, you should file an incident report.

15. _____ Incident reports are meant to protect you, the client, and your agency.

11. Demonstrate ability to use verbal and written information to assist with the care plan

Short Answer.

1. If you are not sure what is important to mention in a care plan meeting, you should:

   _____
   _____
   _____
   _____
   _____
   _____
   _____

2. Why do you think your accurate reporting is so important to the other members of the care team?

   _____
   _____
   _____
   _____

Name: _____

12. Demonstrate effective communication on the telephone

Read the following telephone conversations and think about how the home health aide could have better presented herself on the phone.

Example #1 Leaving a message for the supervisor

Hi, who's this?

Could you get Ms. Crier on the phone, please? I need to talk to her.

She's not there? Do you know where she is? I really have to talk to her right now. My client forgot to take her pill this morning and now she wants to take two and I don't know if that's okay or not, so that's why I need to talk to Ms. Crier.

Okay, well tell her Ella called and have her call me back. Ella. Ella Ferguson. I should be on the schedule.

The number? I don't remember what it is. Let me ask the client.

Okay, the number is 873-9042. I don't know how much longer I'll be here, but have her call me as soon as possible. Bye.

1. What did the home health aide do wrong in this phone conversation?

    _____
    _____
    _____
    _____
    _____
    _____
    _____
    _____

Example #2 Answering calls for the client

Hello? Mrs. Lee? No, she can't come to the phone right now. She's in the bathroom. Who's calling?

And your number?

Can I tell her what this is about?

Okay. I'll give her the message. Goodbye.

2. What did the home health aide do wrong in this phone conversation?

    _____
    _____
    _____
    _____
    _____
    _____
    _____
    _____
    _____

13. Describe cultural diversity and religious differences

Fill in the Blank.

For each sentence, choose the correct term by using the words below. Some words may be used more than once.

Buddhism	Hinduism
Christianity	Islam
Confucianism	Judaism
Agnostic	Atheist

1. Worship at mosques.

    _____

2. Practice religion mostly in China and Japan.

    _____

3. Take communion as a symbol of Christ's sacrifice.

    _____

4. Believe that Allah (God) wants men to follow the teachings of the prophet Mohammed in the Koran.

    _____

5. Religious leaders may be called priests, ministers, pastors, or deacons.

    _____

6. Believe that God gave them laws through Moses and in the Bible, and that these laws should order their lives.

    _____

7. Pray five times a day facing Mecca.

_____

8. This religion started in Asia.

_____

9. May not do certain things, such as work or drive, on the Sabbath.

_____

10. Believe Jesus Christ was the son of God and that he died so their sins would be forgiven.

_____

11. Practice their religion in India and elsewhere.

_____

12. Religious leaders are called rabbis.

_____

13. People who do not deny that God might exist, but they feel there is no true knowledge of God's existence.

_____

14. People who claim that there is no God.

_____

14. List examples of cultural and religious differences

Short Answer.

List three dietary restrictions due to religious beliefs.

1. _____

2. _____

3. _____

15. List ways of coping with combative behavior

Fill in the Blank.

1. Clients may sometimes display

_____

behavior.

2. This behavior may be the result of

_____

affecting the brain, an expression of

_____, or

part of someone's

_____.

3. Do not take such behavior

_____.

4. Always

_____

combative behavior to your supervisor and be sure to

_____ it.

5. It is important for other members of the care team to be

_____ of

this behavior.

16. List ways of coping with inappropriate behavior

Short Answer.

1. List three examples of inappropriate behavior from the client.

_____

_____

_____

_____

_____

_____

_____

2. For each example listed in #1, write down how you should respond to the inappropriate behavior.

_____

_____

_____

_____

_____

_____

_____

5

Infection Control and Standard Precautions

1. Define "asepsis" and explain the chain of infection

Multiple Choice.

1. The following are necessary links in the chain of infection. By wearing gloves, which link is broken, thus preventing the spread of disease?
    a. Reservoir (place where the pathogen lives and grows)
    b. Mode of transmission (a way for the disease to spread)
    c. Susceptible host (person who is likely to get the disease)
    d. Causative agent (the pathogen that causes disease)

2. The following are necessary links in the chain of infection. By getting a vaccination shot for Hepatitis B, which link will be affected and thus prevent you from getting Hepatitis B?
    a. Reservoir (place where the pathogen lives and grows)
    b. Mode of transmission (a way for the disease to spread)
    c. Susceptible host (person who is likely to get the disease)
    d. Causative agent (the pathogen that causes disease)

3. The single most important thing you can do to prevent the spread of disease is to:
    a. Carry dirty linen close to your uniform
    b. Never change your gloves
    c. Remove gloves before cleaning spills
    d. Wash your hands

2. Explain Standard Precautions

True or False.

1. _____ Standard Precautions means treating all blood, body fluids, non-intact skin, and mucous membranes as if they were infected with an infectious disease.

2. _____ Standard Precautions relate to all body fluids except saliva.

3. _____ You can usually tell if someone is infectious by looking at them.

4. _____ The Centers for Disease Control and Prevention defined Standard Precautions.

5. _____ You should wash your hands before putting on gloves.

6. _____ It is okay for you to handle your clients' needles or syringes.

7. _____ Giving mouth care will require you to wear gloves.

8. _____ It is a good idea to wear a mask and protective goggles if you are emptying a bedpan.

9. _____ When cleaning a urinal, you do not need to wear gloves.

Multiple Choice.

10. Standard Precautions should be practiced:
    a. Only on people who look like they have a bloodborne disease
    b. On every single person in your care
    c. Only on people who request that you follow them
    d. Only on people who have tuberculosis

Name: _____

11. Standard Precautions include the following measures:
    a. Washing your hands only before putting on gloves
    b. Wearing gloves if there is a possibility you will come into contact with blood, body fluids, mucous membranes, or broken skin
    c. Touching body fluids with your bare hands
    d. Putting caps on used needles

12. Which of the following is true for Transmission-Based Precautions?
    a. You do not need to practice Standard Precautions if you practice Transmission-Based Precautions.
    b. They are exactly the same as Standard Precautions.
    c. They are practiced in addition to Standard Precautions.
    d. They are never practiced at the same time that Standard Precautions are used.

3. Explain the term "hand hygiene" and identify when to wash hands

True or False.

1. _____ You should wash your hands every time you remove your gloves or any type of PPE.

2. _____ You should only wash your hands on arrival at a client's house, never before you leave it.

3. _____ You do not have to wash your hands if you come into contact with saliva.

4. _____ When working in the kitchen, only wash your hands if you are preparing a meat dish.

5. _____ You should wash your hands after using the restroom.

4. Identify when to use personal protective equipment (PPE)

Short Answer.

Mark an "X" next to the tasks that require you to wear gloves.

1. _____ Handling body fluids

2. _____ Hanging the laundry

3. _____ Potentially touching blood

4. _____ Brushing the client's hair

5. _____ Performing or assisting with perineal care

6. _____ Washing vegetables

7. _____ Putting clean sheets on an unoccupied bed

8. _____ Performing or assisting with mouth care

9. _____ Shaving a client

Word Search.

Complete each of the following sentences and find your answers in the word search.

10. A _____ should be worn when caring for clients with respiratory illnesses.

11. _____ provide protection for your eyes.

12. If there is a chance you could come into contact with _____ membranes or open wounds, you should wear _____ .

13. A mask, glove, goggles, and _____ are all examples of PPE.

q	y	v	f	q	n	m	h	q	i	e	f	c	s
g	l	t	i	f	z	z	u	s	y	w	z	u	v
b	o	b	r	u	h	s	a	e	t	i	o	l	p
k	w	g	b	u	u	r	p	p	t	c	g	q	a
u	d	f	g	q	w	k	j	m	u	d	m	m	t
o	s	l	x	l	n	w	k	m	e	s	t	m	z
y	c	m	c	l	e	n	y	q	i	r	r	k	p
d	x	p	t	t	v	s	w	j	q	i	h	g	p
o	w	q	t	c	a	u	s	o	i	k	s	s	e
o	a	q	k	k	x	y	k	o	g	h	n	r	d
l	o	s	w	q	b	q	p	c	z	e	j	w	a
b	a	q	c	c	c	j	b	c	p	i	d	k	l
m	a	n	y	w	w	y	f	s	j	o	e	o	u
k	i	f	z	f	l	u	i	d	s	v	g	c	l

5. Explain how to handle spills

Short Answer.

Read the following scenario and answer the questions below.

Eddie, a home health aide, takes a urine sample from his client, Mr. Velasquez. When he finishes, he accidentally knocks the container onto the linoleum floor. Some of the urine spills out before he can get to it. Eddie quickly grabs a sponge and begins to wipe up the spill. When he is finished, he finds the mop, puts dishwashing soap into a bucket, and cleans the area again. When he is done mopping, he washes his hands.

Did Eddie follow the proper spill-handling procedure?

_____

If not, what should Eddie have done?

_____
_____
_____
_____
_____
_____
_____
_____
_____

6. Explain Transmission-Based Precautions

Short Answer.

1. List the three categories of Transmission-Based Precautions.

_____
_____
_____

2. Define Airborne Precautions.

_____
_____

_____
_____
_____

3. Define Droplet Precautions.

_____
_____
_____
_____
_____

4. When are Contact Precautions used?

_____
_____
_____
_____

True or False.

5. _____ Family members can use the same dishes as the person who is in isolation.

6. _____ A client in contact or airborne isolation should have a separate bathroom to use.

7. _____ You should wear disposable gloves when handling soiled laundry.

8. _____ Bleach solutions can be used to clean up spills of blood or body fluids and to disinfect surfaces that may have been contaminated.

9. _____ When following isolation procedures, disposable dishes and utensils do not have to be discarded in any particular way.

7. Explain sterilization and disinfection

Short Answer.

1. How does wet heat disinfect? How does dry heat disinfect?

_____
_____
_____
_____

Name: _____

2. What is the difference between sterilization and disinfection?

_____

_____

_____

_____

8. Explain how bloodborne diseases are transmitted

Short Answer.

1. Explain how bloodborne diseases can be transmitted.

_____

_____

_____

_____

_____

_____

_____

_____

_____

_____

2. Name three methods of preventing transmission of bloodborne diseases.

_____

_____

_____

_____

_____

_____

_____

_____

_____

9. Explain the basic facts regarding HIV and hepatitis infection

Fill in the Blank.

1. Hepatitis refers to swelling of the

_____

caused by infection.

2. The major bloodborne diseases in the United States today are

_____ and

_____ .

3. There is no vaccine for hepatitis

_____ .

4. After a number of years, a person with HIV usually develops

_____ .

5. When people are infected with HIV, the disease weakens their

_____ system so that their bodies cannot effectively fight infections.

6. Your employer must offer you a free vaccine to protect you from hepatitis

_____ .

7. The risk of acquiring

_____ is greater than the risk of acquiring

_____ .

8. People with AIDS can lose all ability to fight

_____ and can die from illnesses that a healthy body could handle.

9. Hepatitis

_____ and

_____ are bloodborne diseases that can cause death.

10. Identify high risk behaviors that allow the spread of HIV/AIDS and HBV

True or False.

1. _____ You are at a high risk for HIV/AIDS if you hug an HIV positive person.

2. _____ You can protect against the spread of HIV/AIDS by never sharing used drug needles.

3. _____ Abstinence means having sex with only one person.

4. _____ You are at a high risk for HIV/AIDS if you are having unprotected sex.

5. _____ It may take six months after coming into contact with the virus for an HIV test to show positive.

6. _____ Pregnant women should not get tested for HIV.

7. _____ Having sexual contact with many partners puts you at a high risk for HIV/AIDS.

11. Demonstrate knowledge of the legal aspects of AIDS, including testing

Short Answer.

1. Why may the right to confidentiality be especially important to people with HIV/AIDS?

_____

_____

_____

_____

_____

_____

_____

_____

_____

2. What are two facts regarding HIV testing?

_____

_____

_____

_____

_____

_____

_____

_____

12. Identify community resources and services available to clients with HIV/AIDS

Word Search.

Complete each of the following sentences and find your answers in the word search.

1. There are many resources available for clients who have

_____ or

_____.

2. Meal services,

_____,

and access to experimental

_____ are

all examples of

_____

available to clients with HIV/AIDS.

3. You can check the phone book or the internet for

_____

available in your area.

4. A member of the care team or a

_____

may be able to

_____

services for clients with HIV/AIDS.

n	g	t	j	g	n	i	l	e	s	n	u	o	c
e	e	f	i	c	g	s	e	c	i	v	r	e	s
z	n	t	k	s	d	o	c	b	z	d	z	s	r
z	k	b	a	g	r	u	p	l	l	g	g	e	v
p	a	q	i	n	y	l	x	e	j	u	k	l	o
s	p	e	g	t	i	s	m	h	r	r	y	j	o
e	n	z	q	s	e	d	p	d	o	c	i	m	s
c	g	w	w	f	i	o	r	w	f	e	g	l	x
r	u	g	w	v	s	a	l	o	q	h	s	d	u
u	a	u	g	k	i	a	o	u	o	o	s	y	z
o	b	b	g	d	i	w	z	v	s	c	u	c	o
s	h	w	s	c	l	j	g	w	g	n	h	v	x
e	m	l	o	c	k	x	j	x	s	r	a	i	s
r	w	s	q	q	z	b	q	m	f	l	h	e	v
c	o	m	m	u	n	i	t	y	r	c	i	s	m

13. Explain tuberculosis and list infection control guidelines

Multiple Choice.

1. Tuberculosis may be transmitted:
   a. By coughing
   b. By dancing
   c. By wearing gloves
   d. Through a protective mask

2. Tuberculosis is:
   a. A bloodborne disease
   b. An airborne disease
   c. A non-infectious disease
   d. An untreatable disease

3. Someone with latent TB (TB infection):
   a. Shows symptoms
   b. Falls into a coma almost immediately
   c. Cannot infect others
   d. Can infect others

4. A person with active TB:
   a. Can spread it to others
   b. Does not show symptoms
   c. Cannot eat whole foods
   d. Cannot walk on his or her own

5. TB disease is more likely to develop in people:
   a. Who live near the mountains
   b. Whose relatives had it when they were kids
   c. Whose immune systems are weakened
   d. Who work alone

6. One major factor in the spread of TB is:
   a. Failure to take all the medication prescribed
   b. Following Standard Precautions
   c. Wearing a gown and mask during client care
   d. Following isolation procedures if indicated in the care plan

14. Explain the importance of reporting a possible exposure to an airborne or bloodborne disease

Short Answer.

How do you report possible exposure to an airborne or bloodborne disease?

_____

_____

_____

_____

_____

_____

_____

_____

15. Explain the terms "MRSA," "VRE," and "C. difficile"

True or False.

1. _____ MRSA is spread by direct physical contact.

2. _____ If VRE is established, it is relatively easy to get rid of it.

3. _____ MRSA is spread through indirect contact by touching objects.

4. _____ Handwashing will not help control the spread of MRSA.

5. _____ VRE causes life-threatening infections in people with compromised immune systems.

6. _____ You can help prevent the spread of VRE by washing your hands often.

7. _____ *Clostridium difficile* is a spore-forming bacteria which can be part of the normal intestinal flora.

8. _____ Increasing the use of antibiotics helps lower the risk of developing *C. difficile* diarrhea.

16. List employer and employee responsibilities for infection control

Read the following and mark "er" for employer or "ee" for employee to show who is responsible for infection control.

1. _____ Immediately report any exposure you have to infection.

2. _____ Provide personal protective equipment for use and train how to properly use it.

3. _____ Follow all agency policies and procedures.

4. _____ Take advantage of the hepatitis B vaccination.

5. _____ Provide continuing in-service education on infection control.

6. _____ Establish infection control procedures and an exposure control plan.

7. _____ Follow client care plans and assignments.

8. _____ Participate in annual education programs covering infection control.

6

Safety and Body Mechanics

1. Explain the principles of body mechanics

Labeling.

Complete the illustration by labeling each part with the words listed below.

  alignment
  base of support
  center of gravity
  fulcrum
  lever

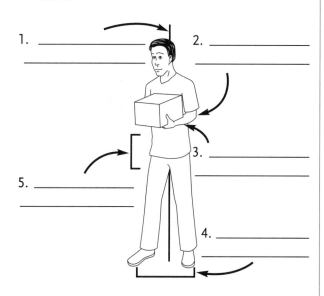

1. _____

   _____

2. _____

3. _____

   _____

5. _____

   _____

4. _____

   _____

2. Apply principles of body mechanics to your daily activities

A.

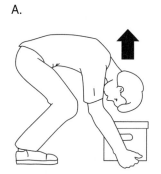

B.

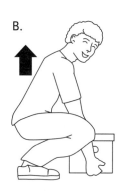

Short Answer.

1. Which picture (A or B) shows the correct way to lift objects? Why is it correct?

    _____

    _____

    _____

    _____

    _____

    _____

Fill in the Blank.

2. When you stand up,

    _____

    with your strong hip and thigh muscles to raise your body and the object together.

3. Bend your

    _____ to
    lower yourself, rather than bending from the _____.

4. Get _____
    whenever possible for lifting or assisting clients.

5. Hold objects

    _____ to
    you when you are lifting or carrying them.

6. Avoid

    _____ at
    the waist. Instead, turn your whole body.

7. If you are making an adjustable bed, adjust the _____
    to a safe working level.

8. Never try to

    _____ a

    falling client.

9. Spread your feet

    _____

    apart and bend your knees when lifting an object from the floor.

10. _____,

    _____, or

    _____

    objects rather than lifting them.

3. List ways to adapt the home to principles of good body mechanics

Multiple Choice.

1. If you cannot reach an object on a high shelf, you should:

    a. Stand on tiptoes to reach it

    b. Use a stepstool

    c. Climb on a counter or lower shelf

    d. Use an umbrella to reach it

2. When sitting for long periods of time, you should not cross your legs because:

    a. It disrupts the alignment of your body

    b. It can wrinkle your clothing

    c. It is unprofessional

    d. You must stand while working

3. To be more comfortable doing tasks that require standing for long periods of time, you can:

    a. Sit down every five minutes

    b. Stand on one foot

    c. Jump up and down

    d. Place one foot on a footrest

4. Frequently-used tools and supplies should be placed

    a. On shelves or counters to reduce the need for bending

    b. On the floor to reduce the need for straining to reach

    c. In boxes where they will be out of the way

    d. In the attic

5. To clean a bathtub, you should:

    a. Bend over

    b. Sit down on the floor

    c. Kneel or use a low stool

    d. Sit inside the tub

4. Identify five common types of accidents in the home

In the following illustrations, circle everything you can find that is wrong in the picture.

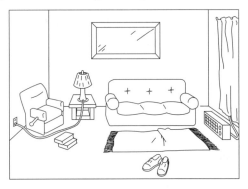

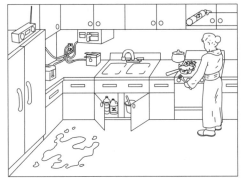

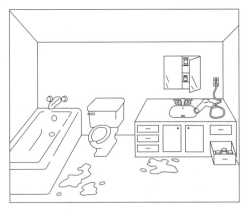

5. List home fire safety guidelines and describe what to do in case of fire

Short Answer.

1. List four things that could be fire hazards.

_____

_____

_____

_____

_____

_____

_____

_____

2. What is important to remember about clothing while working near the stove?

_____

_____

_____

_____

_____

3. How often should you check a smoke alarm? _____

4. RACE stands for:

R: _____

A: _____

C: _____

E: _____

5. PASS stands for:

P: _____

A: _____

S: _____

S: _____

6. List six guidelines for helping clients and family members exit a burning building safely:

_____

_____

_____

_____

_____

_____

_____

_____

_____

6. Discuss the use of restraints and related problems

Short Answer.

1. When can restraints be used?

_____

_____

_____

_____

_____

_____

_____

_____

_____

2. Look at the list of the negative effects of restraint use within this Learning Objective in the textbook. Pick five of the negative effects and for each one you choose, describe why you think restraints could cause those problems.

_____

_____

_____

_____

_____

_____

_____

_____

_____

_____

_____

_____

_____

Name:_____

_____

_____

_____

7. Discuss restraint alternatives and describe what must be done if a restraint is ordered

Short Answer.

1. List five alternatives actions you can take that help reduce the need for a restraint.

   _____
   _____
   _____
   _____
   _____
   _____
   _____
   _____
   _____
   _____

2. Name three types of equipment that can be used instead of restraints.

   _____
   _____
   _____
   _____
   _____

3. The following must be done at regular, ordered intervals whenever a client is in a restraint:

   _____
   _____
   _____
   _____
   _____
   _____
   _____

8. Identify ways to reduce the risk of automobile accidents

Multiple Choice.

1. When driving to a new client's house, you should:
   a. Study the map while driving there
   b. Plan your route before leaving
   c. Look at a map only if you get lost
   d. Talk on your cell phone so that you do not get lonely

2. While driving, it is best to:
   a. Keep your eyes on the road and your hands on the wheel
   b. Listen to music to pass the time
   c. Drive quickly so you will have more time at the client's home
   d. Program your iPod so you do not get bored

3. When backing up in your car, you should:
   a. Only use your rear view mirror
   b. Back up quickly
   c. Turn your head and look behind you
   d. Use your instincts to tell you if someone is behind you

4. Driving at a safe speed means:
   a. Exceeding the speed limit
   b. Making adjustments for road or weather conditions
   c. Driving faster if it is snowing
   D. going 10 miles per hour under the speed limit

5. Seat belts should always be worn because:
   a. They prevent accidents
   b. They help protect you in an accident
   c. They make you look professional
   d. They make it safer to drive much faster

9. Identify guidelines for using your car on the job

True or False.

1. _____ It is not necessary for you to keep track of the miles you drive for work.

2. _____ You should get your car serviced and check the tires regularly.

3. _____ Proof of registration should be kept in your car at all times.

4. _____ Keep proof of insurance at home where it will be safe.

5. _____ Put valuables under a seat or in the trunk if you must leave them in the car.

6. _____ Lock all your doors while driving and when leaving your car.

10. Identify guidelines for working in high-crime areas

Scenarios.

Circle the letter of the answer that best completes the question.

1. You are a home health aide going to visit a client who lives in a high-crime area. You have been to this client's apartment before, but today as you drive up you notice three strange men standing on the sidewalk in front of your client's apartment. They are watching you as you slow down in front of your client's apartment. What do you do?

    a. Ignore them and park your car.

    b. Keep driving past and find a phone or use your cell phone to call your supervisor.

    c. Stop and ask them what they are doing in front of your client's apartment.

    d. Ask them to help you move items from your trunk into the client's house

2. You are getting ready to leave a client's home as it begins to get dark. Your client lives in a large house on a street that is not well-lit. You have parked next to the nearest street light, which is two houses down.

    What should you do on your way to your car?

    a. Run to the car.

    b. Keep your keys inside your purse.

    c. Hold your purse or bag away from your body.

    d. Walk purposefully and confidently.

7

Emergency Care and Disaster Preparation

1. Demonstrate how to recognize and respond to medical emergencies

Crossword.

Across

1. If the person is unable to respond, he may be _____.

5. If the injured person panics, _____to him and tell him what actions are being taken to help him.

8. Make sure you are not in _____.

10. After an emergency, report the _____ only.

Down

2. When you come upon an emergency situation, remain calm, act quickly, and _____ clearly.

3. Notice the _____.

4. Once the emergency is over, you will have to file an _____ report.

6. Falls, _____, and cuts can be emergencies when they are severe.

7. When in doubt, call for _____.

9. Be _____ and confident to help reassure the injured person that he is being taken care of.

2. Describe basic CPR and demonstrate knowledge of first aid procedures

True or False.

1. _____ CPR is an important skill for home health aides to learn.

2. _____ You should perform CPR on an unconscious victim even if you are not properly trained.

3. _____ You can contact the American Heart Association to schedule CPR training.

4. _____ Performing CPR incorrectly cannot further injure a person.

5. _____ Rescue breathing can help in an emergency situation.

6. _____ Brain damage will not occur until 20 minutes after the heart stops beating and the lungs stop breathing.

7. _____ To give a chest compression, you must push in 1 1/2 to 2 inches with each compression.

8. _____ Abdominal thrusts can be used to help someone who is choking.

Name: _____

Multiple Choice.

9. Signs of shock include:
   a. Pale or bluish skin
   b. Lack of thirst
   c. Happiness
   d. Relaxation

10. If you suspect that a client is having a heart attack, you should:
    a. Give him something cold to drink
    b. Loosen the clothing around his neck
    c. Encourage him to walk around
    d. Leave him alone to rest

11. To control bleeding, you should:
    a. Use your bare hands to stop it
    b. Lower the wound below the heart
    c. Hold a thick pad or clean cloth against the wound and press down hard
    d. Give him an aspirin for the pain

12. Which kind of burn involves just the outer layer of skin?
    a. First degree
    b. Second degree
    c. Third degree
    d. Freezer burn

13. Which of the following is NOT a treatment for accidental poisoning?
    a. Ipecac syrup
    b. Activated charcoal
    c. Epsom salts
    d. Ibuprofen

14. To treat a minor burn, you should:
    a. Use ointment
    b. Use grease, such as butter
    c. Use ice water
    d. Use cool, clean water

15. Which of the following is true about assisting a client who is having a seizure?
    a. Give the person a glass of water to drink.
    b. Hold the person down if he or she is shaking severely.
    c. Move furniture away to prevent injury to the person.
    d. Open the person's mouth to move the tongue to the side.

16. If a client faints, you should:
    a. Lower him to the floor
    b. Position him on his side
    c. Elevate his legs one inch
    d. Help him stand up immediately

17. If a client has a nosebleed, what should be your first step?
    a. Report and document the incident.
    b. Apply pressure consistently until the bleeding stops.
    c. Apply a cool cloth on the back of the neck, the forehead, or the upper lip.
    d. Elevate the head of the bed or tell client to remain in a sitting position.

18. If a client falls, you should:
    a. Wait until the end of the day to report the fall
    b. Ask the client to get up so that you can see if she can walk
    c. Look for broken bones
    d. Move the client to the bed

3. Identify emergency evacuation procedures

Short Answer.

List four ways to plan for an evacuation procedure.

_____

_____

_____
_____
_____
_____
_____
_____

4. Demonstrate knowledge of disaster procedures

Multiple Choice.

1. A disaster kit should be assembled before disaster strikes. Disaster supplies include:
   a. An extra set of car keys and a change of clothing
   b. A television set
   c. Cosmetics and a hair dryer
   d. Three pair of shoes

2. In a disaster, stay informed by:
   a. Running out to buy a newspaper
   b. Going outside to find your neighbors
   c. Listening to a radio
   d. Calling your psychic

3. If a disaster is forecast, be prepared by:
   a. Turning off your cell phone
   b. Cleaning your house
   c. Knowing how to start a fire
   d. Wearing appropriate clothing and shoes

4. In the case of tornadoes, you should:
   a. Seek shelter inside, ideally in a steel-framed or concrete building
   b. Hide close to the windows
   c. Stay in a mobile home or trailer
   d. Go outside so that you can see if the tornado is getting closer

5. In the case of lightning, you should:
   a. Find water and stay in the water
   b. Stand by the largest tree you can find
   c. Keep a metal object in your hand
   d. Seek shelter in buildings

6. In the case of floods, you should:
   a. Fill the bathtub with fresh water
   b. Drink water contaminated with flood water to stay hydrated.
   c. Handle electrical equipment
   d. Turn off the gas by yourself

8

Physical, Psychological, and Social Health

1. Identify basic human needs

Short Answer.

1. List six basic physical needs that all humans have.

   _____

   _____

   _____

   _____

   _____

   _____

2. List six psychosocial needs that humans have.

   _____

   _____

   _____

   _____

   _____

   _____

3. Complete your own hierarchy of needs below. Some of the examples have already been completed for you.

   Maslow's Hierarchy of Needs

   Need

   a. Need for self-actualization

   b. Need for self-esteem

   c. Need for love

   d. Safety and security needs

   e. Physical needs

   Example

   a. I need the chance to learn new things.

   b. I need to know that I am doing a good job.

   c. _____

      _____

   d. _____

      _____

   e. _____

      _____

2. Define holistic care

Short Answer.

In your own words, briefly define holistic care.

_____

_____

_____

_____

_____

_____

3. Identify ways to help clients meet their spiritual needs

Mark an "X" next to examples of good ways to assist clients with their spiritual needs.

1. _____ A client tells you that he cannot drink milk with his hamburger due to his religious beliefs. He asks you for some water instead. You take the milk away and bring him some water.

2. _____ A client tells you she is a Baptist and wants to know if you will call the local Baptist church to find out when the next service will be. "A Baptist?" you ask. "Why don't you just attend a Catholic service instead? I'm a Catholic and my church is close by."

Name: _____

3. _____ A client asks you to read a passage from his Bible. He tells you that it will comfort him. You open the Bible and begin to read.

4. _____ A client wants to see a rabbi. You call the rabbi he wants to see.

5. _____ You see a Buddha statue in a client's bedroom. You chuckle and tell the client, "This is kind of funny-looking."

6. _____ A spiritual leader is visiting with a client. You quietly leave the room and shut the door.

7. _____ A client tells you he is Muslim. You begin to explain Christianity to him and ask him to attend a Presbyterian service just to see what it is like.

8. _____ A client tells you that she does not believe in God. You do believe in God but do not argue with her. You listen quietly as she tells you her reasons.

4. Discuss family roles and their significance in health care

Short Answer.

1. List three types of families.

_____

_____

_____

_____

_____

2. What kind of family did you grow up in?

_____

_____

_____

_____

_____

_____

5. Describe personal adjustments of the individual and family to illness and disability

Short Answer.

List three adjustments that family members may need to make due to the client's illness or disability.

_____

_____

_____

_____

_____

_____

_____

6. Identify community resources for individual and family health

Short Answer.

1. If your client or the family asks you for more help, you should:

_____

_____

_____

2. If you think your client or the family needs more help, but they do not ask, you should:

_____

_____

_____

7. List ways to respond to emotional needs of your clients and their families

Short Answer.

1. List three good ways to respond to clients or family members who come to you with problems or needs.

_____

_____

_____

_____

_____

_____

_____

Multiple Choice.

2. You arrive at your client's house to find the wife, Mrs. McNabb, upset and close to tears. She tells you that her husband simply will not eat his breakfast. When you ask what she served him for breakfast, she begins to cry. What is the best thing to do?

    a. Tell her not to cry.

    b. Ask her why she is crying over something so unimportant.

    c. Reassure her that you are here to help.

    d. Tell her that her reaction is probably increasing her stress level.

3. You encourage Mrs. McNabb to talk to you about what is bothering her, and she confesses that she is feeling very overwhelmed. What is the best thing to say to her?

    a. "I know just how you feel. My kids are a handful, too."

    b. "It sounds like you are under a lot of stress. Can I help in some way?"

    c. "Well, I work two jobs myself, and it's no big deal."

    d. "Maybe you should attend church services more often."

4. Mrs. McNabb asks if you can stay longer during your visits to help her out with the cooking and cleaning. What is the best thing to say to her?

    a. "I'll talk to my supervisor and see what she says. Maybe we can work something out."

    b. "You should call a maid service to help you. Here's the phone book."

    c. "I can't do that because I'm a bad cook."

    d. "If you will give me extra money, I may be able to help you."

9

The Human Body in Health and Disease

1. Describe the integumentary system

Fill in the Blank.

1. The largest organ and system in the body is the _____.

2. Skin prevents _____ to internal organs.

3. Skin also prevents the loss of too much _____, which is essential to life.

4. The skin is also a _____ that feels heat, cold, pain, touch, and pressure.

5. Blood vessels _____, or widen, when the outside temperature is too high.

6. Blood vessels _____, or close, when the outside temperature is too cold.

True or False.

7. _____ Pressure sores cannot be prevented.

8. _____ Pressure sores usually occur in areas of the body where bone is close to the skin.

9. _____ The term "shearing" means lubricating dry skin.

10. _____ Another name for pressure sores is decubitus ulcers.

11. _____ Common sites for pressure sores are the chest, nose, and hands.

Labeling.

For each position shown, list the areas at risk for pressure sores.

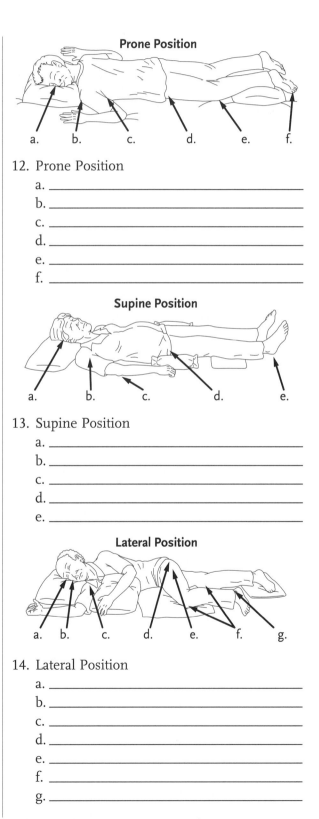

Prone Position

a.   b.   c.   d.   e.   f.

12. Prone Position

    a. _____
    b. _____
    c. _____
    d. _____
    e. _____
    f. _____

Supine Position

a.   b.   c.   d.   e.

13. Supine Position

    a. _____
    b. _____
    c. _____
    d. _____
    e. _____

Lateral Position

a.   b.   c.   d.   e.   f.   g.

14. Lateral Position

    a. _____
    b. _____
    c. _____
    d. _____
    e. _____
    f. _____
    g. _____

Short Answer.

15. List five signs and symptoms to observe and report about the integumentary system.

_____

_____

_____

_____

_____

2. Describe the musculoskeletal system

Short Answer.

1. What can range of motion exercises help prevent?

_____

_____

_____

_____

2. List five of the signs to observe and report about the musculoskeletal system.

_____

_____

_____

_____

_____

Read each of the following. Decide if it is describing a fracture "F", osteoporosis "O", or arthritis "A".

3. _____ Signs and symptoms include low back pain and stooped posture.

4. _____ It occurs most commonly in women after menopause.

5. _____ It is a broken bone.

6. _____ It is the inflammation or swelling of a joint.

7. _____ To treat this, bones are held immobile (by a cast) until the bone can fuse itself back together.

8. _____ This disease causes bone to become porous and brittle.

9. _____ This disease can be prevented by adding extra calcium to the diet.

10. _____ The process of bones fusing back together takes longer with the elderly than with younger people.

3. Describe the nervous system

Crossword.

Across

3. The nervous system also _____ and interprets information from the environment outside the human body.

6. The peripheral nervous system deals with the outer part of the body, via the _____ that extend throughout the body.

Down

1. The nervous system is the _____ center and

2. _____ center of the body.

4. It controls and coordinates all body _____.

5. The central nervous system is composed of the _____ and spinal cord.

Matching.

1. _____ Alzheimer's disease

2. _____ Cerebral palsy

3. _____ CVA or stroke

4. _____ Dementia

5. _____ Epilepsy

6. _____ Multiple sclerosis

7. _____ Parkinson's disease

8. _____ Spinal cord injuries

a. This is an illness in which the myelin sheath that covers the nerves, spinal cord, and white matter of the brain breaks down over time.

b. This is a general term that refers to changes in the brain that alter personality and impair the ability to think and remember.

c. This illness causes a section of the brain to degenerate slowly and progressively.

d. This is a result of an injury to the cerebrum that occurs during pregnancy or the birth process.

e. This is an illness of the brain that produces seizures, which can range in severity from mild to violent.

f. This is an example of dementia with an unknown cause. It cannot be cured, is irreversible, and gets progressively worse.

g. The extent of these depends on the force of the impact and where on the spinal cord the injury is located.

h. This can cause sudden paresis (weakness) or paralysis (immobility) of certain parts of the body.

Short Answer.

9. List eight signs and symptoms to observe and report about the nervous system.

_____

_____

_____

_____

_____

_____

_____

_____

_____

Fill in the Blank.

Fill in the blanks with the words listed below.

cataracts   otitis media

deafness   vertigo

glaucoma

10. _____ is the partial or complete loss of hearing. It can be the result of heredity, disease, or injury.

11. Milky or cloudy spots that develop in the eye and impair vision are _____. They can be surgically removed.

12. Dizziness that is usually the result of an inner ear disturbance or caused by diseases of the brain is _____.

13. _____ is an infection of the middle ear that can be caused by a variety of microorganisms.

14. The condition in which the fluid inside the eyeball is unable to drain, increasing pressure inside the eye and causing damage, is called _____.

Short Answer.

15. List two signs and symptoms to observe and report about the eyes and ears.

_____

_____

_____

_____

4. Describe the circulatory or cardiovascular system

Multiple Choice.

1. The two upper chambers of the heart are called:
   a. Veins
   b. Cells
   c. Left atrium and right atrium
   d. Pericardium

2. During the resting phase, or diastole, of the heart:
   a. Ventricles pump blood through the blood vessels
   b. The heart begins beating rapidly until the next contraction
   c. Circulation stops
   d. The chambers fill with blood

3. Which of the following is one of the functions that the circulatory system performs?
   a. Senses and interprets information from the environment
   b. Supplies food, oxygen, and hormones to cells
   c. Adds waste products to the cells
   d. Processes carbohydrates and proteins

Crossword.

Across

4. Peripheral vascular disease is a disease in which the legs, feet, arms, or hands do not have enough blood

   _____.

Down

1. _____
   is a hardening and narrowing of the blood vessels.

2. Hypertension is also known as

   _____
   _____.

3. Congestive heart failure occurs when the heart is no longer able to _____ effectively.

5. _____ is a squeezing pain or feeling of pressure in the chest, left arm, or jaw.

5. Describe the respiratory system

Fill in the Blank.

1. Respiration is the body taking in
   _____ and removing
   _____.

2. It involves _____
   and _____.

3. The _____
   accomplish this process.

4. _____ is a chronic inflammatory disease. It occurs when the respiratory system is hyper-reactive to irritants, infection, cold air, or allergens such as pollen and dust.

5. _____ is an irritation and inflammation of the lining of the bronchi.

6. _____ is the development of abnormal cells or tumors in the lungs.

7. Symptoms of _____ include coughing, low-grade fever, shortness of breath, and bloody sputum.

8. For most people, _____ can be dealt with by the body's immune system and by rest, fluids, and antibiotics if the infection is bacterial.

9. Two chronic lung diseases are grouped under _____.

10. _____ can be caused by a bacterial, viral, or fungal infection. Acute inflammation occurs in a portion of lung tissue.

Short Answer.

11. List five signs and symptoms to observe and report about the respiratory system.

_____

_____

_____

_____

_____

_____

_____

6. Describe the urinary system

Short Answer.

1. How does urine pass out of the body?

_____

_____

_____

_____

_____

_____

2. What does urine do for the body?

_____

_____

_____

_____

_____

_____

True or False.

3. _____ Cystitis is more common in men.

4. _____ Calculi, or kidney stones, form when urine crystallizes in the kidneys.

5. _____ Kidney dialysis is used for cleaning mucus from the lungs.

6. _____ When someone has a UTI they may experience a painful burning sensation during urination and the frequent feeling of needing to urinate.

7. _____ To avoid infection, women should wipe the perineal area from back to front after elimination.

8. _____ Kidney stones can be the result of a vitamin deficiency or mineral imbalance.

9. _____ Nephritis may cause rusty-colored urine and a decrease in urine output.

10. _____ Excessive salt in the diet can cause damage to the kidneys.

Short Answer.

11. List five signs and symptoms to observe and report about the urinary system.

_____

_____

_____

_____

_____

_____

Name: _____

7. Describe the gastrointestinal system

Crossword.

Across

2. GERD occurs when stomach contents back up into the

   _____.

5. _____
   are enlarged veins in the rectum that cause itching and burning.

7. If heartburn occurs frequently and remains untreated, it can cause scarring or

   _____.

9. Ulcerative colitis is a chronic inflammatory disease of the large

   _____

   that usually occurs in young adults.

10. Raw sores in the stomach or small intestine are called _____

    _____.

13. Treatment of _____ often includes increasing the amount of fiber eaten.

14. To prevent heartburn and GERD, provide an extra pillow to make the client's body more _____ during

    sleep.

Down

1. Surgical treatment of ulcerative colitis may include a _____.

3. Constipation occurs when the feces move too slowly through the intestine as the result of decreased _____ intake and poor diet.

4. Cancer of the gastrointestinal tract is _____ cancer.

6. Heartburn is a result of a weakening of the _____ muscle.

8. A diet of bananas, rice, apples, and tea/toast is called the _____ diet.

11. Clients with peptic ulcers should avoid

    _____.

12. _____ is the frequent elimination of liquid or semi-liquid feces.

Short Answer.

15. List nine signs and symptoms to observe and report about the gastrointestinal system.

    _____

    _____

    _____

    _____

    _____

    _____

    _____

    _____

    _____

8. Describe the endocrine system

Fill in the Blank.

1. Signs and symptoms of diabetes include increased _____ and _____ production.

2. _____ occurs when the thyroid produces too little thyroid hormone and the body processes slow down.

3. Diabetes is a chronic disease that has two major types: _____ and _____.

4. Weight loss, nervousness, and hyperactivity occur with _____.

5. When sugar builds up in the blood and cannot get to the cells, it makes it difficult for the body to process carbohydrates, _____, and proteins.

Short Answer.

6. List eight signs and symptoms to observe and report about the endocrine system immediately.

_____

_____

_____

_____

_____

_____

9. Describe the reproductive system

True or False.

1. _____ Gonorrhea can be treated with antibiotics and is easier to detect in men than in women.

2. _____ People with herpes always experience repeated outbreaks.

3. _____ Condoms can reduce the chances of being infected or passing on some STDs and STIs.

4. _____ Gonorrhea can cause sterility in both men and women.

5. _____ Symptoms of chlamydia include yellow or white discharge from the penis or vagina and a burning sensation during urination.

6. _____ Chlamydia cannot be treated with antibiotics.

7. _____ If left untreated, syphilis can cause brain damage or death.

8. _____ Most women infected with gonorrhea show many early symptoms.

9. _____ Benign prostatic hypertrophy is a fairly common disorder that occurs in both women and men as they age.

10. _____ STDs and STIs can only be transmitted by sexual intercourse.

11. _____ Herpes is caused by a virus and cannot be treated with antibiotics.

12. _____ Chancres, or open sores, that develop on the penis make it easier for syphilis to be detected in men than in women.

13. _____ Penicillin can be used to treat syphilis.

Short Answer.

14. List seven signs and symptoms to observe and report about the reproductive system.

_____

_____

_____

_____

_____

_____

_____

_____

_____

_____

_____

10. Describe the immune and lymphatic systems

Short Answer.

1. What two systems are related to the lymphatic system?

    _____

    _____

    _____

    _____

2. What is lymph?

    _____

    _____

    _____

    _____

3. What is the difference between nonspecific immunity and specific immunity?

    _____

    _____

    _____

    _____

    _____

    _____

4. List three signs and symptoms to observe and report about the immune system.

    _____

    _____

    _____

    _____

10

Human Development and Aging

1. Describe the stages of human development and identify common disorders for each group

Infancy, Birth to 12 Months

True or False.

1. _____ An infant takes three years to be able to move around, communicate basic needs, and feed himself.

2. _____ Infants develop from the hands to the head.

3. _____ Caregivers should encourage infants to stand as soon as they can hold their heads up.

4. _____ Studies show that putting an infant to sleep on its back can reduce the risk of sudden infant death syndrome (SIDS).

Short Answer.

5. List three common disorders of infancy.

_____

_____

_____

_____

_____

_____

Childhood

True or False.

1. _____ Tantrums are common among toddlers.

2. _____ The best way to deal with tantrums is to give the toddler what he wants.

3. _____ Pre-school children are too young to know right from wrong.

4. _____ Children aged three to six are beginning to learn how to play cooperatively with each other.

5. _____ From the ages of six to eight years, most children begin to go through puberty.

6. _____ School-age children develop cognitively and socially.

Short Answer.

7. List three common disorders of childhood.

_____

_____

_____

_____

_____

_____

_____

Adolescence

True or False.

1. _____ Puberty is the stage of growth when secondary sex characteristics, such as body hair, appear.

2. _____ Most adolescents do not struggle with peer acceptance or self-image or self-esteem.

3. _____ Adolescents may be moody due to changing hormones and peer pressure.

4. _____ Eating disorders cannot be life-threatening.

5. _____ Due to changes they are experiencing, adolescents may become depressed and may attempt suicide.

Name: _____

Short Answer.

6. List three common disorders of adolescence.

_____

_____

_____

_____

_____

Adulthood

True or False.

1. _____ By eighteen years of age, most young adults have stopped developing physically, psychologically, and socially.

2. _____ One developmental task that most young adults undertake is to choose an occupation or career.

3. _____ A "mid-life crisis" is a period of unrest when a person has an unconscious desire for change and fulfillment of unmet goals.

4. _____ Middle adults usually do not experience any physical changes due to aging.

5. _____ Menopause is a condition in middle adult women that occurs when the ovaries begin to secrete hormones.

6. _____ By the time a person reaches late adulthood, his or her body has stopped changing due to the effects of aging.

2. Distinguish between fact (what is true) and fallacy (what is not true) about the aging process

True or False.

1. _____ Older adults have different capabilities depending upon their health.

2. _____ As people age, they often become lonely, forgetful, and slow.

3. _____ Diseases and illness are not a normal part of aging.

4. _____ Many older adults can lead active and healthy lives.

3. Discuss normal changes of aging and list care guidelines

Multiple Choice.

1. Older adults experience changes in their skin due to aging because:
   a. Much of the fatty layer beneath the skin is lost
   b. They develop allergies to skin care products
   c. Circulation to the skin is increased
   d. There is not enough moisture in the air

2. Changes to the musculoskeletal system include:
   a. Brittle bones
   b. More flexible joints
   c. Stronger muscles
   d. Increased appetite

3. For clients with poor vision, you should:
   a. Discourage wearing sunglasses outside
   b. Keep eyeglasses clean
   c. Dim the lighting
   d. Have them read a newspaper daily

4. For clients who are hard of hearing, you should:
   a. Speak in a low-pitched voice
   b. Exaggerate your movements as you speak
   c. Shout to be heard
   d. Remove excess earwax

5. For clients with a poor sense of taste and smell, you should:
   a. Check the refrigerator only once a month for spoiled food
   b. Make sure there are working smoke and carbon monoxide detectors in the home
   c. Only feed them spicy foods
   d. Stop performing oral care

6. Which of the following is NOT true about clients who have a poor sense of touch?

   a. Poor sense of touch may be caused by decreased circulation and dry skin.

   b. A client who is confined to bed is at risk for developing pressure sores.

   c. Poor sense of touch can be caused by increased circulation and a greater activity level.

   d. Clients cannot tell if something is too hot. You must be careful with hot drinks and hot water.

7. Clients with heart conditions should:

   a. Exercise vigorously to regain strength

   b. Avoid vigorous activity

   c. Climb stairs as much as possible

   d. Go for long runs when it is hot outside

8. If your client is cold due to poor circulation, the best thing she can do is:

   a. Use a hot water bottle or heating pad

   b. Go without slippers

   c. Wear layers of clothing and turn the thermostat up

   d. Sit in a warm bath most of the day

9. Shortness of breath due to normal aging changes is caused by:

   a. Exercising too hard

   b. Cancer of the lungs

   c. Not exercising enough

   d. Fewer alveoli for oxygen/carbon dioxide exchange

10. Older clients may need to urinate more frequently due to

    a. The bladder not being able to hold as much urine

    b. Drinking more fluids than younger adults

    c. Incontinence

    d. Being thirsty more often

11. Incontinence:

    a. Is a normal part of aging

    b. Could be a sign of illness

    c. Occurs when a person drinks too much fluid

    d. Is always accompanied by constipation

12. Constipation could be the result of:

    a. Faster digestion process due to aging

    b. Eating too much food during the day

    c. Getting too much water or fiber

    d. Slower digestion process due to aging

13. Because the pancreas function lessens due to aging, some clients may:

    a. Develop diabetes

    b. Need to increase fiber intake

    c. Not need a care plan

    d. Develop a poor sense of touch

14. Normal changes in the reproductive system due to aging often result in:

    a. Loss of sexual drive

    b. Thinning of vaginal walls in women

    c. Inappropriate sexual advances

    d. Decrease in the size of the prostate gland in males

15. Which of the following is a result of a weakened immune system due to normal changes of aging?

    a. May take longer to recover from an illness

    b. Developing HIV

    c. Developing anemia

    d. Developing tuberculosis

16. Which of the following is a result of decreased number and size of lymph nodes due to normal changes of aging?

    a. Fewer infections

    b. Less able to contract a fever

    c. Developing diabetes

    d. More infections

17. Insomnia, withdrawal, and moodiness could all be signs of:

    a. Anorexia

    b. Depression

    c. Confusion

    d. Forgetfulness

18. Which of the following would you NOT do to help clients adjust to lifestyle changes due to aging?

    a. Listen to them.

    b. Ensure that their home is safe.

    c. Care about their feelings.

    d. Talk about your own problems to make them forget theirs.

19. What is the most important thing to do if you observe any changes in your client's condition?

    a. Report it to your supervisor.

    b. Report it to your supervisor.

    c. Report it to your supervisor.

    d. All of the above

4. Identify attitudes and living habits that promote good health

Short Answer.

List six things you can do to encourage your clients to stay active, maintain self-esteem, and live independently.

_____

_____

_____

_____

_____

_____

_____

_____

11

Dying, Death, and Hospice

1. Discuss the stages of grief

Multiple Choice.

1. Mrs. Levine, a resident, prays about her terminal illness. She promises God that she will make peace with her sister, whom she has not seen in 20 years, if she is allowed to live. Which stage of dying is Mrs. Levine going through?

   a. Denial

   b. Anger

   c. Bargaining

   d. Depression

   e. Acceptance

2. A terminally ill resident, Mr. Lucero, begins to yell at Peter, his nursing assistant. He says that Peter never took good care of him. He blames Peter for a lack of proper care. Peter does not take it personally because he realizes that Mr. Lucero may be going through the _____ stage of dying.

   a. Denial

   b. Anger

   c. Bargaining

   d. Depression

   e. Acceptance

3. Resident Amy Scott is dying. Her priest visits her at her request. When he asks her if there is anything he can do to help her get things in order, she tells him she has no idea what he is talking about. Instead she begins to tell him the latest news about her son. Mrs. Scott is experiencing:

   a. Denial

   b. Anger

   c. Bargaining

   d. Depression

   e. Acceptance

4. A terminally ill resident, John Calderon, visits with his family. He discusses his funeral arrangements with them. He lets them know that he is concerned about their well-being after he is gone. He says he wants to spend as much time as possible with them before he dies. Mr. Calderon is going through the _____ stage of dying.

   a. Denial

   b. Anger

   c. Bargaining

   d. Depression

   e. Acceptance

5. A terminally ill resident cries constantly. She does not want to talk to anyone. She may be experiencing the _____ stage of dying.

   a. Denial

   b. Anger

   c. Bargaining

   d. Depression

   e. Acceptance

2. Describe the grief process

Word Search.

Complete each of the following sentences and find your answers in the word search.

1. Even if a death is expected, family members and friends may still experience

   _____.

2. When a person dies, family members or friends may cope initially by refusing to believe that they are grieving. This is referred to as _____.

Name: _____

3. Often people experience

_____

about what they did or did not do for the dying person. They may wish they had done more for the dying person.

4. Experiencing _____ towards God, doctors, or even towards the person who died is a normal part of the grief process.

5. Sometimes family members and/or friends may _____ things they said or did not say to a person who has died.

6. Experiencing _____ or depression is very common after a person dies. Missing someone who has died or having a sense of _____ is also a normal part of the grief process.

l	y	g	d	k	o	t	s	l	g	d	z	n	t
o	o	t	p	k	w	e	a	d	a	r	o	l	j
s	w	n	q	o	e	r	d	u	w	i	i	e	u
k	l	z	e	y	i	g	n	o	a	u	n	x	n
b	q	c	x	l	e	e	e	v	g	g	s	e	g
j	m	w	o	l	i	r	s	u	s	e	j	t	d
p	r	l	y	c	f	n	s	w	y	s	v	a	w
e	a	w	c	i	c	f	e	n	t	g	u	k	e
p	a	y	y	o	u	w	s	s	k	c	o	h	s
r	c	e	k	c	r	w	e	u	s	t	m	q	q
d	y	w	l	e	e	s	w	o	w	y	e	z	u
p	z	d	v	z	g	d	v	c	b	v	r	a	b
s	o	a	j	d	n	m	x	b	e	i	t	n	y
u	j	x	h	j	a	b	w	r	s	r	k	j	f

3. Discuss how feelings and attitudes about death differ

Short Answer.

1. Have you ever experienced the death of a loved one? If so, what are some of the emotions you felt?

_____

_____

_____

_____
_____
_____

2. What, if any, religious beliefs do you subscribe to? How do they influence your feelings about death?

_____
_____
_____
_____
_____
_____

3. What cultural background do you have? What cultures are you familiar with? Briefly describe how your culture or other cultures feel about death.

_____
_____
_____
_____
_____
_____
_____

4. Explain common signs of approaching death

Mark an "X" next to the signs of approaching death.

1. _____ Abundance of physical activity

2. _____ Body temperature that is above or below normal

3. _____ Cold, pale skin

4. _____ Disorientation

5. _____ Healthy skin tone

6. _____ Heightened sense of touch

7. _____ Impaired speech

8. _____ Incontinence

9. _____ Perspiration

10. _____ Strong pulse

5. Discuss how to care for a dying client

Crossword.

Across

1. _____
   care means care of the body after death.

3. _____ perspiring clients often.

6. Clients may not be able to communicate that
   they are in _____. Observe
   your clients for signs and report them.

7. Changes of position, back massage,
   _____ care,

8. _____ care, and proper
   body alignment may help to relieve pain.

10. _____
    may be one of the most important things
    you can do for a client who is dying.

Down

2. After death, do not remove any
   _____ or other equipment.

4. _____
   is usually the last sense to leave the body.

5. Observe _____
   to anticipate a client's needs.

9. After a person dies, drainage pads are needed most often under the head and/or under
   the _____.

11. Keep the room _____
    lighted and without glare.

6. Define the goals of a hospice program

True or False.

1. _____ Hospice care can be provided in a
   hospital or in the home.

2. _____ Caregivers should insist that family
   members take breaks.

3. _____ Often, clients who are dying do not
   care about independence anymore.

4. _____ The goals of hospice care are the
   comfort and dignity of the client.

5. _____ It is important in hospice care to
   make clients comfortable, rather
   than keeping an eye to recovery.

Short Answer.

6. Look at the "Dying Person's Bill of Rights"
   on page 131 of your textbook. Pick three
   rights that you feel would be most important
   to you personally. Briefly describe why they
   would be important to you.

_____

_____

_____

_____

_____

_____

_____

Name: _____

7. Identify special skills and attitudes helpful in hospice work

Short Answer.

List five helpful attitudes for hospice work.

_____

_____

_____

_____

_____

_____

_____

_____

_____

_____

2. What are three ways you can take good care of yourself?

_____

_____

_____

_____

_____

_____

_____

_____

_____

_____

8. Describe the role of the hospice volunteer

Fill in the Blank.

1. According to the National Hospice and Palliative Care Organization, approximately _____ hospice volunteers provided care to an estimated _____ people in the U.S. in 2005.

2. Hospice volunteers go through a _____ program to prepare them for hospice work.

3. The services provided by volunteers include caring for the home or family of a dying person, driving or doing errands, and _____ .

9. Discuss the importance of caring for yourself when working in hospice care

Short Answer.

1. How do you alleviate stress in your life?

_____

_____

_____

12

Transfers, Ambulation, and Positioning

1. Explain positioning and describe how to safely position clients

Labeling.

Label each position below and describe comfort measures appropriate for each.

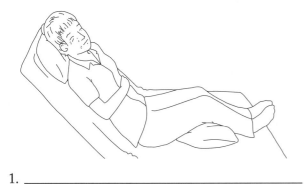

1. _____

Comfort measures: _____

_____

_____

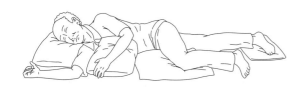

2. _____

Comfort measures: _____

_____

_____

_____

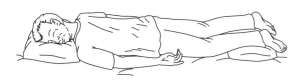

3. _____

Comfort measures: _____

_____
_____
_____
_____

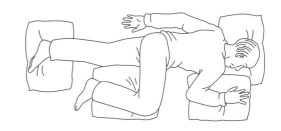

4. _____

Comfort measures: _____

_____

_____

_____

_____

5. _____

Comfort measures: _____

_____

_____

_____

Short Answer.

6. What is shearing?

_____

_____

7. What is logrolling?

_____

_____

Multiple Choice.

8. Before a client who has been lying down moves to a standing position, he should:

   a. Do a few sit-ups in bed to get used to the upright position

   b. Sit up with his feet over the side of the bed for a moment, or dangle

   c. Drink some water or other fluid

   d. Grab a draw sheet

9. To help move a client in bed, you can use a _____ to assist you.

   a. Logroll

   b. Draw sheet

   c. Dangle

   d. Wheelchair

2. Describe how to safely transfer clients

Multiple Choice.

1. Which of the following statements is true of wheelchairs?

   a. Before transferring a client, make sure the wheelchair is unlocked and movable.

   b. Check the client's alignment in the chair after a transfer is complete.

   c. To close a standard wheelchair, turn it upside-down and make the seat flatten.

   d. All clients will need you to transfer them to their wheelchairs.

2. Some clients have a stronger side and a weaker side. The weaker side of the body is called the:

   a. Released side

   b. Separated side

   c. Ambulated side

   d. Involved or affected side

3. When applying a transfer (gait) belt, you should place it:

   a. Around the wheelchair's backrest

   b. Underneath the client's clothing, on bare skin

   c. Over the client's clothing and around the waist

   d. Around your waist so the client can hold on to it

4. The following piece of equipment may be used to help transfer a clients who is unable to bear weight on their legs:

   a. Sling

   b. Slide or transfer board

   c. Wheeled table

   d. Folded blanket

5. Which of the following statements is true of mechanical, or hydraulic, lifts?

   a. You do not need to be trained to use mechanical lifts.

   b. The legs of the stand need to be closed, in their narrowest position, before helping the client into the lift.

   c. Lifts help prevent injury to you and the client.

   d. It is ideal to move clients long distances with mechanical lifts.

3. Discuss how to safely ambulate a client

1. If a client starts to fall, the best thing to do is:

   a. Widen your stance and bring the client's body close to you

   b. Catch the client under the arms to stop the fall

   c. Allow the client to fall since you could be injured trying to break the fall

   d. Let the client fall on top of you to break the fall

2. If a client falls, what is the first thing you should do?

   a. Help the client get up and into bed.

   b. Help the client walk around the room until she is steady.

   c. Call for help if a family member is around.

   d. Have a friend come over so that you can take the client to the hospital together.

3. A client who has some difficulty with balance but can bear weight on both legs should use a:

   a. Walker

   b. Crutch

   c. Wheelchair

   d. Transfer board

4. Ambulation is another word for:

   a. Walking

   b. Movement in a wheelchair

   c. Riding in an ambulance

   d. Logrolling

5. In addition to a transfer (gait) belt, what equipment should you have when you assist a client to ambulate?

   a. Mechanical lift

   b. Rocking chair

   c. Extra pillows

   d. Non-skid shoes

6. If the client is unable to stand without help, you should first:

   a. Hold the client close to your center of gravity

   b. Tell the client to stand on the count of three

   c. Brace the client's lower extremities

   d. Adjust the bed to its highest position

7. When helping a visually-impaired client walk, it is important to:

   a. Keep the client in front of you

   b. Let the client walk beside and slightly behind you

   c. Walk quickly

   d. Avoid mentioning stepping up or down

4. List things you can do to help make your client comfortable

Short Answer.

1. List four things you can do to provide for the comfort and safety of your client in and around the bed.

_____

_____

_____

_____

_____

_____

_____

_____

_____

_____

2. Name two benefits of giving a client a back rub.

_____

_____

_____

_____

_____

_____

3. List five types of positioning devices that can make clients more comfortable and briefly explain the function of each one.

_____

_____

_____

_____

_____

_____

_____

_____

_____

_____

_____

_____

_____

_____

_____

_____

_____

4. What is the purpose of an orthotic device?

_____

_____

_____

_____

_____

13

Personal Care Skills

1. Describe the home health aide's role in assisting clients with personal care

Short Answer.

1. List three things to observe when providing or assisting with personal care.

_____

_____

_____

_____

_____

2. List three things to observe about a client's room after finishing a procedure.

_____

_____

_____

_____

_____

2. Explain guidelines for assisting with bathing

Fill in the Blank.

1. A sturdy, water-resistant chair designed to be placed in the bathtub is called a _____ chair.

2. _____ promotes good health and well-being by removing the perspiration, dirt, oil, and dead skin cells that accumulate on the skin.

3. Before bathing any client or assisting with bathing, make sure the room is _____ enough.

4. The face, hands, _____, and perineum should be washed every day, but com-plete baths or showers can be taken every other day, or even less frequently.

5. A transfer belt, tub chair, and safety bars are all examples of _____ which can make bathing easier and safer.

6. Some agencies only require HHAs to wear gloves during bathing for _____ care or if broken skin is present.

7. _____ or _____ bars are often installed to allow clients something to help them change position.

8. Older skin produces less _____ and oil.

9. Never leave an elderly person or young child _____ while in the bathtub.

10. The bed bath is an excellent time for _____ arms and legs and increasing _____.

3. Describe guidelines for assisting with grooming

True or False.

1. _____ If a client wears regular clothes rather than nightclothes during the day, he or she is more likely to be sleepy.

2. _____ Clients should not choose their clothing for the day; you should pick it for them.

3. _____ Front-fastening bras are easier for clients to manage by themselves.

4. _____ When dressing a client who has a weakness or paralysis on one side, dress the stronger side first.

5. _____ Clients are never embarrassed to have people help them with grooming tasks.

6. _____ You should protect a client's privacy by never exposing more than you need to.

7. _____ If a client has a weaker left arm due to a stroke, refer to it as the "bad" arm.

4. Identify guidelines for good oral care

Short Answer.

1. How often should oral care be performed? When should it be done?

_____

_____

_____

_____

_____

2. List six signs to observe and report about the mouth when performing oral care.

_____

_____

_____

_____

_____

_____

_____

_____

3. What is aspiration?

_____

_____

_____

_____

_____

5. Explain care guidelines for prosthetic devices

True or False.

1. _____ You must submerge a hearing aid in water in order to clean it.

2. _____ Clients should keep an extra battery for their hearing aid on hand.

3. _____ Wearing gloves is unnecessary when caring for an artificial eye.

4. _____ Prostheses are expensive, fitted pieces of equipment.

5. _____ Artificial eyes are held in by a special type of glue.

6. _____ In general, hearing aids should be cleaned daily.

7. _____ A prosthesis is a device that replaces a body part that is missing or deformed because of an accident, injury, illness, or birth defect.

8. _____ Artificial eyes should be rinsed in rubbing alcohol.

9. _____ Eyeglasses are a type of prosthetic device.

10. _____ If a prosthesis is broken or does not fit properly, it is best to try to repair it before reporting it to your supervisor.

6. Explain guidelines for assisting with toileting

Labeling.

Label each assistive device below and explain its purpose.

Name: _____

1. _____

Purpose: _____

_____

_____

_____

2. _____

Purpose: _____

_____

_____

3. _____

Purpose: _____

_____

_____

_____

4. _____

Purpose: _____

_____

_____

_____

7. Describe how to dispose of body wastes

Short Answer.

1. How must washcloths used to clean perineal areas be washed?

_____

_____

_____

_____

2. Why must you wear gloves when handling bedpans, urinals, or basins that contain wastes, including dirty bath water?

_____

_____

_____

_____

_____

_____

14

Core Healthcare Skills

1. Explain the importance of monitoring vital signs

Short Answer.

1. What can changes in vital signs indicate? Which changes should be immediately reported to a supervisor?

_____

_____

_____

_____

_____

_____

_____

2. What are the four sites for measuring body temperature?

_____

_____

_____

3. Name seven conditions that indicate you should not take the person's temperature orally.

_____

_____

_____

_____

_____

_____

_____

Labeling.

For each of the mercury-free thermometers shown below, write the temperature reading to the nearest tenth degree.

4. _____

5. _____

6. _____

7. _____

Multiple Choice.

8. Which of the following is the normal temperature range for the oral method?

   a. 96.6 - 98.6 degrees F

   b. 93.6 - 97.9 degrees F

   c. 98.6 - 100.6 degrees F

   d. 97.6 - 99.6 degrees F

9. Which of the following blood pressures falls within the normal range?

   a. 119/75

   b. 135/90

   c. 91/70

   d. 140/80

Name: _____

10. Which of the following thermometers is used to take a temperature from the ear?

   a. Oral thermometer

   b. Rectal thermometer

   c. Axillary thermometer

   d. Tympanic thermometer

11. Which of the following thermometers is used to take a temperature from the armpit?

   a. Oral thermometer

   b. Rectal thermometer

   c. Axillary thermometer

   d. Tympanic thermometer

12. Which temperature is considered to be the most accurate?

   a. Oral

   b. Rectal

   c. Axillary

   d. Tympanic

13. Why are mercury-free thermometers considered safer than the mercury thermometers?

   a. They do not contain mercury, which is a dangerous and toxic substance.

   b. They are smaller than mercury thermometers.

   c. They are read differently than mercury thermometers.

   d. They are less expensive than mercury thermometers.

14. If you must use a mercury thermometer, the best way to clean it is:

   a. Put in the dishwasher.

   b. Wash it with soap and hot water.

   c. Wipe it from stem to bulb with an alcohol wipe.

   d. Spray it with glass cleaner and wipe it with a paper towel.

15. How long do digital thermometers take to display a person's temperature?

   a. 2 to 60 seconds

   b. 1 to 2 minutes

   c. 3 minutes

   d. Less than 1 second

16. Where is the apical pulse located?

   a. Underneath a person's chin

   b. On the inside of the wrist

   c. On the inside of the elbow

   d. On the left side of the chest, just below the nipple

Short Answer.

17. What is the most common site for monitoring the pulse?

_____

_____

_____

True or False.

18. _____ An unusually high or low pulse rate does not necessarily indicate disease.

19. _____ A rapid pulse may result from dehydration or shock.

20. _____ It is best to measure the apical pulse on infants and small children because their pulse points are harder to find.

21. _____ The apical pulse is heard by listening directly over the wrist.

Fill in the Blank.

22. Breathing air into the lungs is also called

_____.

23. Exhaling air out of the lungs is also called

_____ .

24. The normal respiration rate for adults ranges from

_____ to

_____ breaths

per minute.

25. The normal respiration rate for infants ranges from

_____ to
_____ breaths per minute.

Short Answer.

26. Why is it important to observe your client's respirations without letting him or her know that is what you are doing?

_____

_____

_____

_____

_____

Matching.

For each of the following terms, write the letter of the correct definition from the list.

27. _____ 100–119 mmHg

28. _____ 60–79 mmHg

29. _____ diastolic phase

30. _____ hypertension

31. _____ hypotension

32. _____ mmHg

33. _____ sphygmomanometer

34. _____ systolic phase

a. Blood pressure in the arteries when the heart is contracting

b. Low blood pressure

c. Blood pressure in the arteries when the heart is relaxed

d. High blood pressure

e. Blood pressure cuff

f. Normal range for diastolic blood pressure

g. Measuring unit used for blood pressure

h. Normal range for systolic blood pressure

Short Answer.

35. What questions should you ask to get the most accurate information if a client complains of pain?

_____

_____

_____

_____

_____

_____

_____

_____

36. List five measures to reduce a client's pain.

_____

_____

_____

_____

_____

_____

_____

_____

_____

_____

37. Name ten signs and symptoms of pain that should be reported to your supervisor.

_____

_____

_____

_____

_____

_____

_____

_____

_____

_____

_____

_____

2. List three types of specimens you may collect from a client

Short Answer.

1. List the three types of specimens you may have to collect from a client.

   _____

   _____

   _____

   _____

   _____

2. Which type of specimen may require a 24-hour collection?

   _____

   _____

   _____

3. What is a "hat"?

   _____

   _____

   _____

4. What is another term for "calculi"?

   _____

   _____

   _____

5. What is a clean catch urine specimen, and what is its purpose?

   _____

   _____

   _____

   _____

   _____

6. When is the best time of day to collect sputum?

   _____

   _____

3. Describe the importance of fluid balance and explain intake and output (I&O)

Short Answer.

1. A healthy person generally needs to take in about 64 to 96 oz. of fluid each day. How many mL is this? _____ to _____ mL. How many cups is this?

   _____ to _____ cups.

2. Mrs. Wyant drinks half of a glass of orange juice. You know that the glass holds about 1 cup of liquid. How many mL of orange juice did Mrs. Wyant drink?

   _____

3. Mr. Bernicke just ate some chocolate pudding from a 6 oz. container. You measure the leftover pudding, which is about 35 mL. How many mL of pudding did Mr. Bernicke eat? _____

4. Miss Cahill has a bowl of soup for lunch. The soup bowl holds about 1 ½ cups of liquid. Convert this to mL. _____. Miss Cahill finishes most of her soup, but there is about 25 mL left. How many mL of soup did Miss Cahill eat?

   _____

5. List three guidelines to follow when a client vomits.

   _____

   _____

   _____

   _____

   _____

4. Describe the guidelines for catheter care

Short Answer.

1. Briefly define an indwelling catheter.

   _____

   _____

_____
_____
_____
_____
_____

2. Briefly define an external or condom catheter.

_____
_____
_____
_____
_____
_____

3. List three guidelines to follow when working around clients with catheters.

_____
_____
_____
_____
_____
_____
_____
_____
_____

4. List six things to report to the supervisor about a client's catheter.

_____
_____
_____
_____
_____
_____
_____
_____

5. Explain the benefits of warm and cold applications

Crossword.

Across

4. Report to your supervisor if you observe excessive _____ or pain.

6. _____ or numbness with warm or cold applications are other signs to report to your supervisor.

Down

1. Heat relieves _____ and muscular tension.

2. Increased _____ brings more oxygen and nutrients to the tissues for healing.

3. Cold applications help to bring down high _____.

5. Another type of heat application is a warm soak of the perineal area, which is also called a _____.

6. Cold applications can help stop _____ and reduce swelling.

Multiple Choice.

7. Which of the following is a type of dry heat application?
    a. Cold compress
    b. Warm tub bath
    c. Warm soak
    d. Disposable warm pack

Name: _____

8. Heat relieves pain by:

   a. Reducing swelling and increasing blood flow

   b. Decreasing oxygen to the tissues

   c. Bringing down high fevers

   d. Causing numbness

9. Which of the following is a type of moist cold application?

   a. Warm sitz bath

   b. Warm compress

   c. Disposable cold pack

   d. Ice pack

10. What is the proper water temperature when you are making a warm compress?

   a. 105 to 110 degrees Fahrenheit

   b. 90 to 99 degrees Fahrenheit

   c. 100 to 104 degrees Fahrenheit

   d. 101 to 105 degrees Fahrenheit

6. Explain how to apply non-sterile dressings

Short Answer.

What is the difference between sterile and non-sterile dressings?

_____

_____

_____

_____

_____

_____

_____

_____

_____

7. Describe the purpose of elastic stockings and how to apply them

Short Answer.

What is the purpose of elastic stockings?

_____

_____

_____

_____

_____

_____

_____

_____

_____

_____

_____

_____

8. Define the term "ostomy" and list care guidelines

True or False.

1. _____ An ostomy is an operation to create an opening from an area inside the body to the outside.

2. _____ A stoma is an artificial opening in the abdomen through which stool is eliminated.

3. _____ In a colostomy, the stool will generally be semi-solid.

4. _____ In an ileostomy, the stool will generally be solid.

Short Answer.

5. Why do you think a client with an ostomy might feel embarrassed about it?

_____

_____

_____

_____
_____
_____
_____

Multiple Choice.

6. How often should an ostomy bag be emptied and cleaned or replaced?

   a. Once a day

   b. Every hour

   c. Whenever a stool is eliminated

   d. Before a client wakes up

7. What could cause a food blockage?

   a. Too much liquid in the client's diet

   b. A large amount of high-fiber food in the client's diet

   c. Skin irritation

   d. Cold compresses

9. Describe how to assist with an elastic bandage

Multiple Choice.

1. Elastic bandages are also known as:

   a. Non-sterile bandages

   b. Plastic bandages

   c. Liquid bandages

   d. Aseptic bandages

2. One purpose of elastic bandages is to:

   a. Elevate a cast

   b. Hold a dressing in place

   c. Cover pressure sores

   d. Help with ambulation

3. Apply elastic bandages snugly enough to control _____ and prevent movement of _____.

   a. Temperature, the client

   b. Bleeding, dressings

   c. Elevation, dressings

   d. Movement, temperature

4. How soon should an HHA check on a client after applying a bandage?

   a. One hour

   b. The next day

   c. Five hours

   d. 15 minutes

15

Rehabilitation and Restorative Care

1. Discuss rehabilitation and restorative care

Short Answer.

1. List four goals of a rehabilitative program.

_____

_____

_____

_____

_____

2. Rehabilitation will be used for many of your clients, but particularly for those who have suffered what three incidents?

_____

_____

_____

3. What kind of care usually follows rehabilitation, and what is its goal?

_____

_____

_____

_____

_____

2. Explain the home care rehabilitation model

Short Answer.

List five members of the team who may participate in a client's restorative care.

_____

_____

_____

_____

3. Describe guidelines for assisting with restorative care

True or False.

1. _____ You should downplay any setbacks a client experiences so he or she does not become discouraged.

2. _____ Your reactions and attitudes really do not affect a client's progress.

3. _____ If you can do a task faster than your client, you should do it yourself.

4. _____ Do not report any decline in a client's ability.

5. _____ Family members and clients will take cues from you on how to behave.

6. _____ Tasks are less overwhelming when they are broken down into small steps.

7. _____ It is important to report any signs of depression or mood changes in a client.

4. Describe how to assist with range of motion exercises

Matching.

For each of the following terms, write the letter of the correct definition from the list below.

1. _____ active assisted range of motion

2. _____ active range of motion

3. _____ contracture

4. _____ passive range of motion

5. _____ range of motion

a. The permanent and often painful stiffening of a joint and muscle, caused by immobility

b. Exercises performed by the client with some assistance and support

c. Exercises used by clients who are not able to move on their own

d. Exercises that put a particular joint through its full arc of motion

e. Exercises performed by the client himself, using his own muscle power

Labeling.

For each of the following illustrations, put the correct term of the exercise.

6. _____

7. _____

8. _____

9. _____

10. _____

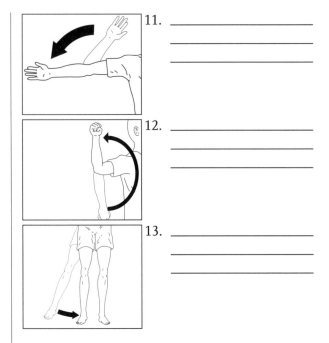

11. _____

12. _____

13. _____

5. Explain guidelines for maintaining proper body alignment

Fill in the Blank.

1. Observe principles of _____. Remember that proper alignment is based on a straight _____.

    _____ or rolled or folded _____ may be needed to support the small of the back and raise the knees or head in the supine position.

2. Keep body parts in natural _____. In a natural hand position, the fingers are slightly _____. Use _____ to keep covers from resting on feet in the supine position.

3. Prevent external rotation of _____. Change _____ frequently to prevent muscle stiffness and pressure ulcers. Every _____ hours is usually adequate.

6. List important observations to make about changes in a client's skin

Short Answer.

1. List eight important observations to make about changes in a client's skin.

_____

_____

_____

_____

_____

_____

_____

_____

_____

_____

_____

2. List the four accepted stages of pressure sores, including a brief description of what the sore looks like at each stage.

_____

_____

_____

_____

_____

_____

_____

_____

_____

_____

_____

3. What are four changes to ebony complexions that might indicate injury to the tissue?

_____

_____

_____

_____

_____

_____

7. List guidelines for providing basic skin care and preventing pressure sores

Crossword.

Across

4. Reposition immobile clients at least every _____ hours.

3. Provide regular care for skin to keep it _____ and

6. _____.

5. A _____, chamois skin, or bed pad, absorbs moisture under the back and buttocks.

7. Avoid pulling the client across sheets during transfers or repositioning because it causes

_____.

Down

1. _____ the skin frequently, using light, circular strokes to increase circulation.

4. Keep the bottom sheet _____ and free from wrinkles and the bed free

2. from _____.

5. Report changes you observe in a client's

_____.

Multiple Choice.

8. When complete baths are not given or taken every day, how often should you check the client's skin or provide skin care?
   a. Daily
   b. Twice per month
   c. Three times a day
   d. Four times a week

9. How often should you reposition an immobile client?
   a. Three times a day
   b. At least every two hours
   c. Twice a day
   d. Every 15 minutes

10. What purpose does a bed cradle have?
    a. As a liner for chairs or wheelchairs
    b. To absorb moisture
    c. To keep top sheets from rubbing the client's skin
    d. To make a bed or chair softer

8. Describe the guidelines for caring for clients who have fractures or casts

Multiple Choice.

1. When caring for a client who has a cast, _____ the extremity that is in a cast to help stop swelling.
   a. Lower
   b. Double bandage
   c. Elevate
   d. Shake

2. Keep the cast _____ at all times.
   a. Dry
   b. Wet
   c. Hot
   d. Pointed

3. Osteoporosis occurs more frequently in _____ people.
   a. Young
   b. Active
   c. Elderly
   d. Diabetic

4. A bone must be _____ to allow the fusion of fractured parts.
   a. Lowered
   b. Surgically repaired
   c. Wet
   d. Immobilized

5. Signs and symptoms of a fracture include:
   a. Heat
   b. Cold
   c. Swelling
   d. Dryness

6. Fractures are broken bones and may be caused by:
   a. Eating too much fiber
   b. Talking
   c. Osteoporosis
   d. Laughing

7. You can place a wet cast on _____ so that its shape is not altered as it dries.
   a. A metal surface
   b. Pillows
   c. Concrete
   d. A wood floor

8. When can a client insert something inside the cast?
   a. When skin itches
   b. After the cast dries
   c. When the cast is wet
   d. Never

9. List the guidelines for caring for clients who have hip fractures

True or False.

1. _____ Most fractured hips require surgery.

2. _____ You should provide ROM exercises for a leg on the side of a hip replacement when you feel it is necessary.

3. _____ A hip fracture is not really a serious injury.

4. _____ Elderly people heal slowly.

5. _____ Home health aides may disconnect traction assembly.

6. _____ A client recovering from a hip replacement should not sit with his or her legs crossed. The hip cannot be at less than a 90-degree angle.

7. _____ Dress a client recovering from a hip replacement starting with the unaffected side first.

8. _____ A red or warm incision after hip replacement surgery must be reported to the supervisor.

Multiple Choice.

9. What is the main reason that hip fractures are more common in the elderly?

   a. Bones weaken as people age.

   b. Elderly people get too much exercise.

   c. Elderly people are depressed.

   d. Elderly people can bear more weight on their bones.

10. Which side should clients recovering from hip replacements dress first?

   a. Affected side

   b. It does not matter.

   c. Unaffected side

   d. Left side, no matter which side is affected

11. What does "PWB" stand for?

   a. Previously weakened bones

   b. Partial weight bearing

   c. Patient's weight before

   d. Patient wants baths

12. If you see "NWB" on a client's care plan, the client:

   a. Can support 100 percent of his or her body weight on one leg

   b. Can support some weight, but not all, on one or both legs

   c. Is unable to support any weight on one or both legs

   d. Can use stairs without assistance

10. List ways to adapt the environment for people with physical limitations

Short Answer.

Choose an adaptive device from Figure 15-31 in the textbook that you did not choose for the Chapter Review. Describe how it might help a client who is recovering from or adapting to a physical condition.

_____

_____

_____

_____

_____

_____

_____

_____

11. Identify reasons clients lose bowel or bladder control

Word Search.

Complete each of the following sentences and find your answers in the word search.

1. When people cannot control the muscles of the bowel or bladder, they are said to be

   _____.

2. A _____ placed over a protective sheet can help absorb moisture and protect the client's skin from the rubber or plastic.

3. Clients who are incontinent need to be kept

   _____,

   _____,

   and free from odor.

4. Offer incontinent clients a

   _____ frequently.

5. Bathing and good _____ help keep urine and feces from irritating the skin.

6. Clients who have lost

_____ or
_____ con-
trol need reassurance and understanding.

e	k	i	a	t	f	u	u	y	e	x	n	r	n
z	g	i	p	e	t	b	s	j	r	c	a	j	x
l	w	g	f	e	e	x	o	d	a	d	e	k	k
u	w	j	k	h	q	d	h	l	c	g	l	f	j
q	q	i	o	s	p	j	q	h	l	s	c	m	g
b	a	a	d	w	o	l	d	a	a	t	q	h	l
l	l	v	q	a	b	f	l	c	e	v	b	l	k
o	e	a	w	r	r	e	y	i	n	m	e	f	s
k	m	w	d	d	y	r	p	x	i	x	d	b	f
h	z	g	o	d	d	p	p	g	r	d	p	x	v
d	w	v	x	b	e	n	a	t	e	o	a	v	r
g	p	c	z	f	l	r	p	p	p	o	n	a	h
t	n	e	n	i	t	n	o	c	n	i	s	w	m
b	d	t	u	s	r	t	a	n	w	m	g	y	s

12. Explain the guidelines for assisting with bowel or bladder retraining

Fill in the Blank.

1. Encourage the client to eat foods that are high in _____.

2. Wear _____ when handling body wastes.

3. Encourage the client to drink plenty of

_____.

Do this even if urinary incontinence is a problem.

4. Never show _____
   or _____
   toward clients who are incontinent. The problem is out of their control.

5. Offer _____
   words for successes or even attempts to control bladder and bowels.

6. Do not _____
   the client.

7. Assist your client with good

_____.

This prevents skin breakdown and promotes proper hygiene.

13. Describe the benefits of deep breathing exercises

Short Answer.

What can deep breathing exercises help?

_____

_____

_____

_____

_____

_____

_____

_____

16

Medications and Technology in Home Care

1. List four guidelines for safe and proper use of medications

True or False.

1. _____ Home health aides must never handle or administer medications unless specifically trained and assigned to do so.

2. _____ Home health aides are not allowed to touch the client's medication containers in any way.

3. _____ It is not important for the home health aide to know what medications the client is taking.

4. _____ Home health aides should report any symptoms, such as dizziness, stomachache, or vomiting, because these could indicate a side effect or drug interaction.

5. _____ Aspirin and ibuprofen are examples of over-the-counter drugs.

2. Identify the five "rights" of medications

Word Search.

List each of the five "rights" of medications below, and then find them in the word search.

1. The right _____

2. The right _____

3. The right _____

4. The right _____

5. The right _____

```
e  b  g  q  k  d  x  m  c  q  r  w  u  k
i  f  a  c  i  i  m  e  h  d  z  t  v  q
g  n  t  o  n  o  f  d  t  l  i  t  b  i
t  c  x  p  u  j  j  i  u  m  v  n  k  m
o  l  d  g  w  z  p  c  e  b  f  r  j  h
b  i  u  k  g  g  f  a  j  y  q  z  k  c
u  e  c  w  o  w  j  t  q  x  e  q  j  d
l  n  j  f  w  p  c  i  s  q  x  p  w  k
g  t  a  p  m  l  h  o  a  m  o  u  n  t
i  p  f  y  z  e  b  n  r  a  y  q  t  t
t  f  i  h  q  l  f  b  e  o  k  v  f  c
t  n  w  a  m  e  w  p  k  t  u  n  v  i
i  x  q  i  h  d  r  g  v  c  l  t  i  n
f  p  m  l  t  o  i  e  b  g  t  n  e  w
```

3. Explain how to assist a client with self-administered medications

True or False.

1. _____ All medications should be taken with food to avoid stomach irritation.

2. _____ To avoid any problems with drug interactions, you should document every medication the client takes, whether it is part of the treatment plan or not.

3. _____ Sedatives should never be mixed with alcohol.

4. _____ You can remind a client when it is time to take medication.

5. _____ Allergic reactions to medication may require emergency intervention.

Name: _____

Short Answer.

6. List seven ways in which you may help clients with self-medication.

_____
_____
_____
_____
_____
_____
_____
_____
_____
_____

7. List ten things involving self-medication that HHAs are NOT allowed to do.

_____
_____
_____
_____
_____
_____
_____
_____
_____
_____

8. Name five common side effects that clients may experience from their medication.

_____
_____
_____
_____
_____
_____
_____

4. Identify observations about medications that should be reported right away

Short Answer.

1. What should you do if your client shows signs of a reaction to a medication or complains of side effects?

_____
_____
_____

2. What should you do if your client takes medication in the wrong amount, at the wrong time, or takes the wrong kind of medication?

_____
_____
_____

5. Describe what to do in an emergency involving medications

Scenarios.

1. Mrs. Mallory takes several prescription medications each day as ordered by her physician. On the day you are scheduled to visit her, you arrive at her home to find Mrs. Mallory sitting down in a chair and looking very ill. When you ask her if she is okay, she tells you that she feels very sick to her stomach and she thinks she might faint. Mrs. Mallory says that she might have taken too much medication, because she could not remember if she had already taken her morning dosage. What should you do?

_____
_____
_____
_____
_____
_____

2. You arrive at Mr. MacIntyre's home at 8:30 a.m. and find him lying in bed. You are unable to wake him, and then you notice several bottles of pills on the table next to the bed. They are all open, and some of the pills are scattered on the table and the floor. What do you do?

_____

_____

_____

_____

_____

_____

_____

6. Identify methods of medication storage

True or False.

1. _____ The client's medication should be kept separate from medicine used by other members of the household.

2. _____ If young children or confused adults are present in the home, medications should be stored on top of the refrigerator where they cannot be reached.

3. _____ Store all medications away from heat and light, as appropriate.

4. _____ If medication has expired, you should discard it in the trash.

7. Identify signs of drug misuse and abuse and know how to report these

Multiple Choice.

1. Proper medication usage includes which of the following?

    a. Refusing to take medications

    b. Mixing medication with alcohol

    c. Taking illegal drugs

    d. Taking the proper dose at the right time

2. The best thing to do if your client refuses to take medication is:

    a. Push the client to take the medication, explaining that it is good for him or her

    b. Try to find out why the client does not want to take the medication and report to the supervisor

    c. Call 911 for emergency medical help

    d. Call the client's doctor immediately

3. A common reason why people avoid taking prescribed medication is:

    a. They dislike the side effects.

    b. They are stubborn.

    c. They do not want to feel better.

    d. They would rather get well without it.

4. Signs of drug misuse or abuse include:

    a. Increased appetite and weight gain

    b. Unusual cheerfulness

    c. Depression, moodiness, or anorexia

    d. Better relationships with family members

5. The drugs that pose the highest risk for causing drug dependency are:

    a. Pain medications and tranquilizers

    b. Antihistamines (allergy medicine)

    c. Beta blockers

    d. Multivitamins

8. Demonstrate an understanding of oxygen equipment

Fill in the Blank.

1. Some clients with breathing difficulties may receive _____. It is more _____ than what we breathe in the air. You should never stop, adjust, or _____ oxygen for a client.

2. Some clients receive oxygen through a _____.

3. Clients who do not need concentrated oxygen all the time may use a _____ when they need oxygen.

4. Oxygen can be irritating to the nose and mouth. Wash and dry skin carefully, and provide frequent _____ care. Offer the client plenty of _____.

5. Oxygen is a dangerous fire hazard because it supports _____.

Multiple Choice.

6. Who is responsible for servicing oxygen tanks or concentrators in a client's home?
    a. The doctor who prescribed the oxygen
    b. The HHA
    c. The client's family members
    d. The agency that supplies the oxygen

7. When is it acceptable for you stop, adjust, or administer a client's oxygen?
    a. Whenever the client requests that you do so
    b. Every three days
    c. According to the care plan
    d. Never

8. What is a cannula used for?
    a. To provide nitrogen to the client
    b. To lock a wheelchair in place
    c. To provide concentrated oxygen through a client's nose
    d. To secure a face mask to a client who only occasionally needs oxygen

9. Liquid oxygen can cause which of the following?
    a. Frostbite
    b. Drug abuse or misuse
    c. Digestive problems
    d. Sterile water

10. What kind of water is used in humidifying bottles for oxygen concentrators?
    a. Sparkling water
    b. Purified water from natural springs
    c. Sterile water
    d. Tap water

11. What is the purpose of a humidifier?
    a. To put only warm moisture in the air
    b. To remove moisture from the air
    c. To put warm or cool moisture in the air
    d. To clean the air without adding moisture

9. Explain guidelines for the care of a client with an IV

Short Answer.

Briefly describe your only responsibility when caring for a client with an IV.

_____

_____

_____

_____

_____

_____

17

Clients with Disabilities

1. Identify common causes of disabilities

Short Answer.

1. List three factors that affect how well a person copes with a disability.

_____

_____

_____

_____

_____

2. List six diseases and disorders that may cause disability.

_____

_____

_____

_____

_____

3. What are two types of disabilities that can be caused by injury to the head or spinal cord?

_____

_____

_____

2. Describe daily challenges a person with a disability may face

Short Answer.

List five daily challenges a person with a disability may face.

_____

_____

_____

_____

_____

_____

3. Define terms related to disabilities and explain why they are important

Short Answer.

1. What are some terms you use to define yourself (i.e. race, sexual orientation, religion)? Why?

_____

_____

_____

_____

_____

_____

_____

_____

_____

_____

_____

2. List a few terms that you think would be a more preferable way to refer to people with disabilities.

_____

_____

_____

_____

4. Identify social and emotional needs of persons with disabilities

Fill in the Blank.

1. Basic social and emotional needs include independence, social interaction, a sense of worth, and _____.

2. Treat all clients with _____.

3. Do not push clients beyond their _____.

4. Give clients _____ to show you what they can do by themselves.

5. Explain how a disability may affect sexuality and intimacy

True or False.

1. _____ A disabled person does not generally experience sexual desires.

2. _____ For disabled people, the ability to meet sexual needs may be limited.

6. Identify skills you have already learned that can be applied to clients with disabilities

Short Answer.

List three skills you have already learned that can be applied to working with clients with disabilities.

_____

_____

_____

_____

_____

7. List five goals to work toward when assisting clients who have disabilities

Fill in the Blank.

1. Promote self-care and _____.

2. Assure the client's _____.

3. Promote the client's health and _____.

4. Maintain the client's _____ and self-worth.

5. Maintain the _____ of the client's household.

Short Answer.

6. Why is it a good idea to think about how you might feel if you had a disability when working with clients with disabilities?

_____

_____

_____

_____

_____

_____

_____

_____

_____

_____

8. Identify five qualities of excellent service needed by clients with disabilities

Short Answer.

List the five qualities of excellent service needed by clients with disabilities.

_____

_____

_____

_____

_____

_____

_____

9. Explain how to adapt personal care procedures to meet the needs of clients with disabilities

True or False.

1. _____ When dealing with a blind client, identify yourself immediately when you enter a room.

2. _____ Avoid touching people with cerebral palsy.

3. _____ Usually people with ALS eventually have to breathe and be fed with the assistance of ventilators and tubes.

4. _____ Quadriplegia refers to the loss of function of the muscles in arms, chest, and lower body.

5. _____ Symptoms of MS include blurred vision, tremors, poor balance, and difficulty walking.

6. _____ When dealing with hearing impaired clients, it is easier if you pretend you understand what they are saying even if you do not.

7. _____ Multiple sclerosis is usually not diagnosed until late adulthood.

8. _____ People with muscular dystrophy do not live past childhood.

9. _____ A person with Parkinson's disease is at a high risk for falls.

10. _____ Activities that require excessive effort should not be pursued by people who have cerebral palsy.

11. _____ Children who have Down syndrome do not appear physically different from any other child.

12. _____ Head injuries may cause paresis, which means that the entire body is affected.

13. _____ Spina bifida cannot cause brain damage.

14. _____ Rehabilitation is not necessary for clients with spinal cord injuries.

15. _____ Disabilities caused by ALS or Lou Gehrig's disease begin with muscle weakness in the limbs or throat.

16. _____ Signs of hearing loss include speaking loudly and responding inappropriately.

17. _____ Speech impairment is one effect of cerebral palsy.

18. _____ A person with Parkinson's disease may have tremors or shaking. This makes it very difficult for him or her to perform ADLs such as eating and bathing.

19. _____ You may be trained to help clients in using a prosthesis when they have had a body part amputated.

20. _____ Cataracts can be corrected with surgery.

21. _____ Emotional support is a very important part of rehabilitation for a head or spinal cord injury.

22. _____ It is a good idea to use an imaginary clock when explaining the position of objects to a visually impaired client.

23. _____ It is possible that some babies born with spina bifida will be able to walk and experience no lasting disabilities.

24. _____ Braille is a fast and easy-to-learn method for blind clients to communicate.

25. _____ Phantom sensation after an amputation is not real. Ignore clients if they mention it.

26. _____ Glaucoma is a cause of blindness.

27. _____ When dealing with a hearing impaired client, you should shout to be heard.

Multiple Choice.

28. The four degrees of mental retardation are mild, moderate, severe, and _____.

    a. Independent

    b. Prolonged

    c. Profound

    d. Physical

29. In which of the following ways can home health aides help a developmentally disabled client?

    a. Teaching the client how to drive

    b. Performing all the client's ADLs

    c. Teaching the client self-care and assisting with ADLs

    d. Ignoring the individual needs of the client

30. If a client has muscular dystrophy, his or her legs may be:

    a Strong and limber

    b. Weak and stiff

    c. Muscular

    d. Quadriplegia

31. Multiple sclerosis is a progressive disease that affects the:

    a. Central nervous system

    b. Respiratory system

    c. Lymphatic system

    d. Circulatory system

32. The ability to see objects in the distance better than objects nearby is called:

    a. Nearsightedness

    b. Cataracts

    c. Glaucoma

    d. Farsightedness

10. List important changes to report and document for a client with disabilities

Short Answer.

1. What should you do if you notice a client is unable to perform a task that he or she was previously able to do?

    _____

    _____

    _____

2. Give two examples of emotional changes that should be observed and reported.

    _____

    _____

    _____

    _____

18

Mental Health and Mental Illness

1. Identify five characteristics of mental health

Short Answer.

1. Define mental health.

_____

_____

_____

_____

_____

2. List five characteristics of a person who is mentally healthy.

_____

_____

_____

_____

_____

_____

_____

2. Identify four causes of mental illness

True or False.

1. _____ Signs and symptoms of mental illness include confusion, disorientation, agitation, and anxiety.

2. _____ A situation response may be triggered by severe changes in the environment.

3. _____ A mentally healthy person cannot experience a situation response.

4. _____ Mental illness can be brought on by substance abuse or a chemical imbalance.

5. _____ The building blocks of mental health are self-respect and self-worth.

6. _____ Traumatic experiences early in life do not cause mental illness.

7. _____ Mental illness cannot be inherited.

8. _____ Extreme stress may result in mental illness.

3. Distinguish between fact and fallacy concerning mental illness

True or False.

1. _____ A fallacy is a false belief.

2. _____ People who are mentally ill have the power to control their illness.

3. _____ People who are mentally ill do not want to get well.

4. _____ Mental illness is a disease just like any physical illness.

5. _____ People who are mentally ill often cannot control their emotions or responses to people and situations.

4. Explain the connection between mental and physical wellness

Short Answer.

Briefly describe why mental health is important to physical health.

_____

_____

_____

_____

_____

5. List guidelines for communicating with mentally ill clients

Labeling.

Fill in the blanks to show how to practice good communication skills with mentally ill clients.

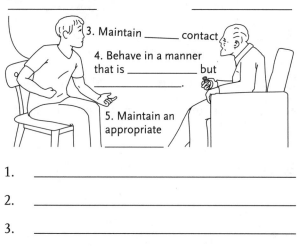

1. Stand or sit with a posture that says you're _____

2. Practice _____

3. Maintain _____ contact

4. Behave in a manner that is _____ but _____ .

5. Maintain an appropriate

1. _____
2. _____
3. _____
4. _____
5. _____

6. Identify and define common defense mechanisms

Multiple Choice.

1. Which of the following is NOT true about defense mechanisms?

   a. They help to release tension.

   b. They help a person cope with stress.

   c. People who are mentally ill use them to a greater degree than people who are not.

   d. They help a person understand his or her emotional problems and behaviors.

2. Telling your co-worker "Let's throw spitballs at our boss" is an example of which kind of defense mechanism?

   a. Displacement

   b. Regression

   c. Rationalization

   d. Projection

3. A co-worker gets the promotion that you have wanted for a long time. When your friend asks you if you are upset, you say, "No, not at all." This is an example of:

   a. Denial

   b. Displacement

   c. Regression

   d. Projection

7. Describe the symptoms of anxiety, depression, and schizophrenia

Fill in the Blank.

Using the words below, complete each of the following statements. Each word is used only once.

anxiety	major
apathy	manic
claustrophobia	obsessive compulsive
delusions	phobia
hallucinations	schizophrenia

1. Lack of interest in activities is called _____ .

2. An intense form of anxiety, such as fear of flying, is called a _____ .

3. Illusions that a person sees or hears are called _____ .

4. When a person washes his hands over and over again as a way of dealing with anxiety, this type of behavior is called _____ disorder.

5. _____ is uneasiness or fear, often about a situation or condition.

6. _____ depression may cause a person to lose interest in everything he once cared about.

7. Fear of being in a confined space, such as an elevator, is called _____ .

8. _____ is a brain disorder that affects a person's ability to think and communicate clearly.

9. _____ depression causes a person to swing from profound depression to extreme activity.

10. _____ are persistent false beliefs, such as thinking that other people can read one's thoughts.

8. Explain how medications can help a client who is mentally ill

True or False.

1. _____ Mental illness cannot be treated.

2. _____ Medication and psychotherapy are commonly used to treat mental illness.

3. _____ You will be responsible for giving mentally ill clients their medication.

4. _____ Medication can allow the mentally ill to function more completely.

9. Explain your role in caring for clients who are mentally ill

Short Answer.

List four special responsibilities that you will have when caring for mentally ill clients.

_____

_____

_____

_____

_____

_____

_____

10. Identify important observations that should be made and reported

True or False.

1. _____ It is important to report to your supervisor if a mentally ill client stops taking medication.

2. _____ You do not need to worry about a mentally ill client discussing suicide if he or she is just joking about it.

3. _____ You should report to your supervisor if a mentally ill client has an extremely happy reaction to bad news.

11. List the signs of substance abuse

Multiple Choice.

1. Circle all of the following substances that can be abused:
   a. Alcohol
   b. Cigarettes
   c. Decongestants
   d. Diet aids
   e. Illegal drugs
   f. Glue
   g. Paint
   h. Prescription medicine

2. Your client has been acting a little strangely lately. She gets upset very easily and her eyes are always red. She does not eat much, and sometimes you can smell alcohol on her breath, even in the morning. What should you do?
   a. Confront your client about what you have noticed.
   b. Call Alcoholics Anonymous.
   c. Document your observations and report them to your supervisor.
   d. Search the client's cabinets for alcohol and throw away whatever you find.

19

New Mothers, Infants, and Children

1. Explain the growth of home care for new mothers and infants

True or False.

1. _____ Most new mothers stay in the hospital for several days to a week after childbirth.

2. _____ Bed rest is ordered if a woman shows signs of early labor.

3. _____ Home care aides are called upon to help when an expectant mother is put on bed rest by her doctor.

4. _____ New mothers today are generally more energetic when they come home than women in the past.

5. _____ Bed rest may help prevent labor from starting before the baby is ready to be born.

6. _____ Natural childbirth has been increasing in popularity.

2. Identify common neonatal disorders

Short Answer.

List three common neonatal disorders.

_____

_____

_____

_____

_____

_____

_____

3. Identify ways of assisting a new mother with her transition to the home

Fill in the Blank.

Use this list of words and phrases to fill in the blanks in the following sentences.

caesarean section   housekeeping

care plan   monitor

diapering   support

episiotomy   bathing

feeding

1. An incision sometimes made in the perineal area during vaginal delivery is an

   _____.

2. Since each situation is different, what you do to care for the new mother will be spelled out in the

   _____.

3. Basic care for the baby includes

   _____,

   _____, and

   _____.

4. You may be required to do light

   _____ to help

   the new mother.

5. A birthing procedure in which the baby is delivered through an incision in the mother's abdomen is called a

   _____.

6. You may be asked to

   _____ the

   equipment if the baby is receiving oxygen.

7. More care may be required depending on how much

   _____ the

   mother has from her family or others.

Name: _____

4. List important observations to report and document

Short Answer.

Document the following scenario.

You arrive at your client's house at 8 a.m. to care for baby Eric, a two-day-old newborn, and find the house dirty, the new mother Anne in a sitz bath, and baby Eric in the crib crying. The mother is also crying and complains of getting "no sleep last night." What course of action should you take? How would you document this?

_____
_____
_____
_____
_____
_____
_____
_____
_____
_____
_____
_____
_____

5. Explain guidelines for safely handling a baby

Labeling.

Label the type of hold shown in each figure.

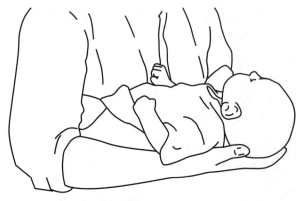

1. _____

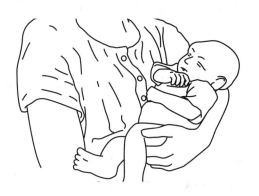

2. _____

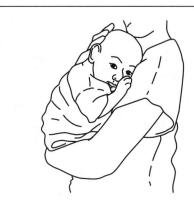

3. _____

6. Describe guidelines for assisting with feeding a baby

Multiple Choice.

1. If the baby does not latch onto the nipple right away, the mother should stroke his:

   a. Toes

   b. Elbows

   c. Cheek

   d. Forehead

2. Many professionals recommend that mothers try breastfeeding for _____ week(s) before deciding whether to continue or stop.

   a. Five

   b. Ten

   c. One

   d. Two

3. Powdered formula is sold in:

   a. Bottles

   b. One- or two-pound cans

   c. Sterilized pitchers

   d. Covered plastic bowls

4. The cheapest formula is usually:
   a. Ready-to-feed
   b. Concentrated liquid
   c. Powdered
   d. Prepared

5. A good position for breastfeeding is:
   a. Lying face down on the bed
   b. Sitting upright in a comfortable chair
   c. Rocking rapidly in a chair
   d. Bending over the crib

6. What food should the mother not eat because it affects breast milk?
   a. Chocolate
   b. Fruit
   c. Yogurt
   d. Fish

7. Before feeding, check the temperature of the formula on your wrist. It should feel:
   a. Warm
   b. Hot
   c. Cold
   d. Frozen

8. The mother can break the suction of a nursing baby by:
   a. Pulling down the baby's ears
   b. Putting her finger in the baby's mouth
   c. Sucking on the baby's toes
   d. Shaking the baby

9. Which of the following is best for bottle-fed newborns?
   a. Whole milk
   b. Special infant formula
   c. 1/2 and 1/2
   d. Skim milk

7. Explain guidelines for bathing and changing a baby

True or False.

1. _____ You should wear disposable gloves when changing or bathing a baby.

2. _____ You should dry a baby's head immediately after washing his hair.

3. _____ Test a baby's bath temperature by dipping the baby's hand in it to see if it turns red.

4. _____ Moisture contributes to diaper rash.

5. _____ It is okay to have both hands off the baby if it is only for a minute.

6. _____ Children generally wear diapers until they are 8 to 12 months old.

7. _____ Newborns will need between six and ten diaper changes in 24 hours.

8. _____ Always use baby powder after giving a baby a bath.

9. _____ If a newborn baby has a loose bowel movement with every feeding, you should be concerned.

10. _____ Babies should be changed frequently to avoid diaper rash.

8. Explain guidelines for special care

Matching.

For each of the following terms, write the letter of the correct definition from the list below.

1. _____ apnea

2. _____ circumcision

3. _____ oxygen

4. _____ rubbing alcohol

5. _____ umbilical cord

a. The cord that connects the baby to the placenta

b. Used for care of the umbilical cord stump to prevent infection

c. Given to some babies who have breathing problems; it is extremely flammable

d. The removal of part of the foreskin of the penis

e. The state of not breathing

9. Identify special needs of children and describe how children respond to stress

Short Answer.

1. List some examples of physical needs that children have.

   _____

   _____

   _____

   _____

   _____

2. List an example of a mental need that children have.

   _____

   _____

   _____

3. List some examples of emotional needs that children have.

   _____

   _____

   _____

   _____

   _____

4. List five reasons that children may experience stress.

   _____

   _____

   _____

   _____

   _____

5. List five factors that influence the way in which children respond to stress.

   _____

   _____

   _____

   _____

   _____

   _____

   _____

6. In what ways might school-age children react to stress?

   _____

   _____

   _____

   _____

   _____

   _____

7. In what negative ways might adolescents react to stress?

   _____

   _____

   _____

   _____

   _____

10. List symptoms of common childhood illnesses and the required care

Fill in the Blank.

1. Cleaning, disinfection, and _____ are the best ways to control infection.

2. Infant acetaminophen is _____ than children's acetaminophen, and the dosage is much smaller.

3. Frequent loose or watery bowel movements are called _____.

4. Children with diarrhea may experience _____, thus doctors may recommend electrolyte-replacement drinks.

5. In general, children should not be given _____, because it has been associated with some serious disorders.

6. The BRAT diet consists of bananas, rice, applesauce, and

   _____.

7. Treatment of a fever includes a lukewarm bath or _____.

8. _____ foods, such as pasta or crackers are usually allowed when children have diarrhea.

9. Rest and _____ are recommended for fevers.

10. Too much acetaminophen can cause _____ damage.

11. Identify guidelines for working with children

Scenarios.

Read the following scenarios and decide how to respond.

1. Patrick and his older brother Greg have just returned home from school. Patrick is upset because he did not win a prize for his science project, but his brother did. He cried at school, and some of the other kids made fun of him. He becomes visibly distressed again as he relates this story to you. How can you respond to Patrick?

   _____

   _____

   _____

   _____

   _____

   _____

   _____

   _____

2. You notice that Doug has been withdrawn all afternoon. He did not go outside to play after school, and at dinner, he refuses to eat anything. He makes comments like "nobody cares about me." What are some things you can do?

   _____

   _____

   _____

   _____

   _____

   _____

   _____

   _____

   _____

   _____

12. List the signs of child abuse and neglect and know how to report them

Short Answer.

1. Psychological abuse includes:

   _____

   _____

   _____

   _____

2. Sexual abuse includes:

   _____

   _____

   _____

   _____

3. Child neglect is:

   _____

   _____

   _____

20

Common Chronic and Acute Conditions

1. Define arthritis and identify treatments and care guidelines

Short Answer.

1. What does arthritis mean?

_____

_____

_____

2. List five common treatments for arthritis.

_____

_____

_____

_____

_____

_____

_____

3. List five care guidelines for arthritis.

_____

_____

_____

_____

_____

_____

_____

_____

_____

2. Define cancer and list eight risk factors for cancer

Fill in the Blank.

Fill in the blanks with the words listed below.

benign   malignant

cancer   tumor

cure

1. _____ is a general term used to describe many types of malignant tumors.

2. A _____ is a cluster of abnormally growing cells.

3. _____ tumors grow slowly in local areas and are considered non-cancerous.

4. _____ tumors grow rapidly and invade surrounding tissues.

5. There is no known _____ for cancer.

3. List the warning signs of cancer

Short Answer.

Mark an "X" beside the American Cancer Society's warning signs of cancer.

1. _____ Change in bowel or bladder habits

2. _____ Difficulty breathing

3. _____ Dizziness

4. _____ Thickening or lump in breast

5. _____ Memory loss

6. _____ Obvious change in wart or mole

7. _____ Pain or swelling of the joints

8. _____ Persistent hoarseness

9. _____ Persistent indigestion or difficulty swallowing

10. _____ Nausea or vomiting

11. _____ Sweet, fruity breath odor

12. _____ Sore that does not heal

13. _____ Unusual bleeding or discharge from body opening

14. _____ Headache

4. Identify common treatments for cancer

Multiple Choice.

1. The key treatment for malignant tumors of the skin, breast, bladder, colon, rectum, stomach, and muscle is:

   a. Surgery

   b. Chemotherapy

   c. Radiation

   d. Herbal remedies

2. Nausea, vomiting, diarrhea, hair loss, and decreased resistance to infection are all side effects of which treatment?

   a. Surgery

   b. Chemotherapy

   c. Diet and exercise

   d. Herbal remedies

3. This treatment method uses drugs to destroy cancer cells and limit the rate of cell growth:

   a. Surgery

   b. Chemotherapy

   c. Radiation

   d. Herbal remedies

4. This treatment method involves removing as much of the tumor as possible to prevent cancer from spreading:

   a. Surgery

   b. Chemotherapy

   c. Radiation

   d. Herbal remedies

5. This treatment method kills normal and abnormal cells in a limited area, sometimes causing skin to become sore, irritated, or burned.

   a. Surgery

   b. Chemotherapy

   c. Radiation

   d. Herbal remedies

5. Describe care guidelines for the client who has cancer

Multiple Choice.

1. To help promote good nutrition, you can do the following:

   a. Use metal utensils for clients

   b. Serve favorite foods that are high in nutrition

   c. Restrict nutritional supplements

   d. Serve foods with little nutritional content

2. If your client is experiencing pain, you should:

   a. Assist with comfort measures

   b. Not report it

   c. Give the client pain medication

   d. Tell the client that you cannot do anything about it

3. In providing skin care, which of the following is NOT a good idea?

   a. Use lotion regularly on dry or delicate skin.

   b. Remove markings that are used in radiation therapy.

   c. Offer back rubs for comfort and circulation.

   d. Do not apply lotion to areas receiving radiation therapy.

4. Which of the following is NOT a good idea when providing oral care?

   a. Rinsing with commercial mouthwash

   b. Using a soft-bristled toothbrush

   c. Assisting client to brush and floss regularly

   d. Being gentle when giving oral care

5. Which of the following is a good idea for communicating with a client who has cancer?

   a. Insist that the client tell you what he or she is going through.

   b. Tell the client about any new medications that he or she should take.

   c. If the client is worried, tell him or her "It'll all be fine."

   d. Listen to the client if he or she feels like talking.

6. You are caring for Mrs. Brady, a client who has cancer. Mrs. Brady has a lot of visitors, and most of them call before they come over. One visitor has a habit of stopping by whenever she happens to be in the area, and today she has come at a very bad time for Mrs. Brady. What should you tell this visitor?

   a. "Mrs. Brady enjoys your visits, but unfortunately this is not a good time for her. Perhaps you can give her a phone call later on. I'll certainly let her know you were here."

   b. "Mrs. Brady can't just drop whatever she is doing to speak with you. You should call before you come over."

   c. "Most people know that it is very inconsiderate to stop by someone's house without calling first."

   d. "Lady, I'm just the caregiver. It's not my fault if Mrs. Brady doesn't want to see you."

6. Identify community resources available to people with cancer and their families

Short Answer.

List three types of organizations that provide services and support for people with cancer and their families.

_____

_____

_____

7. Describe diabetes and identify its signs and complications

Short Answer.

1. What causes diabetes?

_____

_____

_____

_____

_____

2. List three signs and symptoms of diabetes.

_____

_____

_____

_____

_____

Multiple Choice.

3. Diabetes can lead to the following complications:

   a. Reduced circulation

   b. Mastectomy

   c. Cancer

   d. Arthritis

4. Changes in the circulatory system from diabetes can cause:

   a. Hair loss

   b. Heart attack and stroke

   c. Opportunistic infections

   d. COPD

5. The most common form of diabetes is:

   a. Type 1 diabetes

   b. Type 2 diabetes

   c. Pre-diabetes

   d. Gestational diabetes

6. Poor circulation and impaired healing may result in:
   a. Urinary tract infections
   b. Cancer
   c. Gangrene
   d. AIDS

7. Gangrene can lead to:
   a. Loss of bowel control
   b. Paralysis
   c. Congestive heart failure
   d. Amputation

8. What type of diabetes occurs when a person's blood glucose are above normal but not high enough for a diagnosis of Type 2 diabetes?
   a. Gestational diabetes
   b. Type 1 diabetes
   c. Pre-diabetes
   d. Hyperglycemia

9. Good _____ care is vitally important for people with diabetes.
   a. Foot
   b. Hair
   c. Facial
   d. Mouth

8. Describe the differences between insulin reaction and diabetic ketoacidosis, and list care for each

Matching.

For each of the following statements, decide whether it describes insulin reaction or diabetic ketoacidosis. Then write "I" for insulin reaction or "D" for diabetic ketoacidosis.

1. _____ This is also known as hypoglycemia.

2. _____ This is also called hyperglycemia.

3. _____ This can result from too much food.

4. _____ This can result from too little food.

5. _____ Dry skin is a sign.

6. _____ Perspiration is a sign.

7. _____ Blurred vision is a sign.

8. _____ Flushed cheeks are a sign.

9. _____ Nausea and vomiting are a sign.

10. _____ Abdominal pain is a sign.

11. _____ Numbness of the lips and tongue is a sign.

12. _____ Confusion is a sign.

13. _____ Sweet, fruity breath odor is a sign.

14. _____ Cold, clammy skin is a sign.

9. List care guidelines for the client with diabetes

True or False.

1. _____ Meals must be eaten at the same time every day for the client with diabetes.

2. _____ If your client is not following her diet, report this to your supervisor.

3. _____ Encourage the client with diabetes to eat as many carbohydrates as possible.

4. _____ Exercise has not been shown to help clients with diabetes.

5. _____ Home care aides are not permitted to inject insulin.

6. _____ Check the expiration date on insulin before giving it to the client.

7. _____ All states require that home health aides test a diabetic client's blood and urine every day for sugar or insulin levels.

8. _____ A small sore on a diabetic client can be dangerous.

9. _____ Home health aides should never cut any client's toenails, but especially not a diabetic client's toenails.

10. _____ Diabetics should go barefoot.

10. Describe a meal plan for the client with diabetes

Short Answer.

Design a sample meal plan that follows the Sample Meal Plan on page 289 in the textbook and uses foods from the Exchange List Sample Items, also in the same box.

Breakfast:

_____

_____

_____

_____

Snack:

_____

_____

_____

_____

Lunch:

_____

_____

_____

_____

Snack:

_____

_____

_____

Dinner:

_____

_____

_____

_____

Snack:

_____

_____

_____

_____

_____

11. Define cerebral vascular accident (CVA) and list common warning signs

Crossword.

Across

1. _____ is weakness on one side of the body.

4. A warning sign of a CVA is _____.

6. It is the result of a lack of _____ in the brain.

7. A stroke is caused when the blood supply to the brain is cut off suddenly by a _____ or a ruptured blood vessel.

Down

2. Expressive _____ is the inability to speak or to speak clearly.

3. Another name for cerebral vascular accident is a _____.

5. _____ is paralysis on one side of the body.

12. Describe six common physical changes in CVA clients

Short Answer.

Mark an "X" next to the physical changes listed below that a client who has had a stroke may experience.

1. _____ confusion
2. _____ decreased circulation
3. _____ developing pressure sores
4. _____ receptive aphasia
5. _____ difficulty breathing
6. _____ dysphagia
7. _____ hallucinations or delusions
8. _____ inability to speak
9. _____ increased thirst and hunger
10. _____ loss of sensations such as temperature or touch
11. _____ loss of cognitive abilities
12. _____ loss of bowel or bladder control
13. _____ memory loss
14. _____ night sweats
15. _____ persistent hoarseness or a nagging cough
16. _____ poor judgment
17. _____ restlessness
18. _____ one-sided neglect
19. _____ wandering
20. _____ weakness on one side of the body

13. Describe care guidelines and communication techniques for the CVA client

True or False.

1. _____ Clients with paralysis or loss of movement do not need physical therapy.

2. _____ Range-of-motion exercises strengthen muscles and keep joints mobile.

3. _____ Leg exercises improve circulation.

4. _____ When helping with transfers or ambulation, stand on the client's stronger side.

5. _____ Always use a gait belt for safety.

6. _____ Refer to the side that has been affected by stroke as the "bad" side.

7. _____ Gestures and facial expressions are important in communicating with the CVA client.

8. _____ Clients who suffer confusion or memory loss due to a stroke may feel more secure if you establish a routine of care.

9. _____ CVA clients are not at risk of falling.

10. _____ Clients with a loss of sensation could easily burn themselves.

11. _____ For safety purposes, unnecessary clutter and throw rugs should be removed.

12. _____ Pay close attention to changes in the skin of the CVA client, and observe for skin breakdown.

13. _____ Let the client do things for him- or herself whenever possible.

Scenarios.

Read each of the following statements, and answer the questions.

14. Jody, a home health aide, is getting ready to prepare lunch for Mr. Elliot, who is recovering from a stroke. Mr. Elliot has difficulty communicating and also suffers from confusion. "Let's see," Jody says. "For lunch we can have soup, sandwiches, some leftover casserole, or I can make a salad. Now, what would you like to eat?" What is wrong with the way Jody is communicating with Mr. Elliot?

_____

_____

_____

_____

_____

_____

15. Mr. Elliot's wife comes home after running some errands and asks how her husband is doing. As she and Jody walk into the kitchen where Mr. Elliot is sitting, Jody says, "Mr. Elliot is having trouble today with his eating. Just look at him. He's spilled all over himself." What is wrong with what Jody has just said?

_____

_____

_____

_____

_____

_____

_____

16. Jody notices that Mr. Elliot seems to be having trouble saying words clearly. He is beginning to get frustrated because he cannot tell Jody what he wants. Jody decides to ask only yes or no questions, so she tells Mr. Elliot, "If you find it too difficult to speak right now, why don't you try nodding your head for "yes" and shaking your head for "no"." What is Jody doing right?

_____

_____

_____

_____

_____

_____

_____

_____

Fill in the Blank.

17. When assisting with a transfer for a client with one-sided weakness, always lead with the _____ side.

18. Dress the _____ side first. This prevents unnecessary bending.

19. Undress the _____ side first.

20. _____ equipment is used to help the client dress himself.

21. When assisting a CVA client to eat, place the food in the client's

_____.

14. Identify common circulatory disorders, their symptoms, and care guidelines

Matching.

For each of the following terms, write the letter of the correct definition from the list below.

1. _____ angina pectoris

2. _____ atherosclerosis

3. _____ congestive heart failure

4. _____ diuretics

5. _____ dyspnea

6. _____ hypertension

7. _____ myocardial infarction

8. _____ nitroglycerin

a. difficulty breathing

b. the condition in which the heart fails to pump effectively, causing blood to back up into the heart instead of circulating

c. another name for chest pain, pressure, or discomfort

d. another name for high blood pressure

e. medication that relaxes the walls of the coronary arteries

f. a condition in which blood flow to the heart muscle is blocked and the muscle cell dies

g. drugs that reduce fluid in the body

h. a hardening and narrowing of the blood vessels

15. Define COPD and list care guidelines

Multiple Choice.

1. Clients with COPD have difficulty with:
   a. Breathing
   b. Urination
   c. Maintaining weight
   d. Vision

2. A constant fear of a person who has COPD is:
   a. Constipation
   b. Incontinence
   c. Not being able to breathe
   d. Heart attack

3. A client with COPD should be positioned:
   a. Lying flat on his back
   b. Sitting upright
   c. Lying on his stomach
   d. Lying on his side

4. Your role in caring for a client with COPD includes:
   a. Being calm and supportive
   b. Adjusting oxygen levels
   c. Making changes in the client's diet
   d. Doing everything for the client as much as possible

5. Chronic bronchitis and emphysema are grouped under:
   a. Chronic obstructive pulmonary disease, or COPD
   b. Muscular dystrophy, or MD
   c. Hypertension, or HTN
   d. Coronary artery disease, or CAD

16. Define HIV and AIDS and describe care guidelines

True or False.

1. _____ HIV and AIDS are the same thing.

2. _____ HIV can only be transmitted sexually.

3. _____ The first stage of HIV infection involves symptoms similar to flu.

4. _____ There is no known cure for AIDS.

5. _____ AIDS dementia complex occurs in the early stages of AIDS.

Short Answer.

6. List five signs and symptoms of HIV infection and AIDS.

   _____

   _____

   _____

   _____

   _____

7. What is an opportunistic infection?

   _____

   _____

   _____

   _____

   _____

Multiple Choice.

8. Care for the person with AIDS should focus on:
   a. Helping to find a cure for HIV
   b. Preventing visits from friends and family
   c. Providing relief of symptoms and preventing complications
   d. Making judgments about the client

9. If your client with AIDS has a poor appetite, you should:
   a. Give them an over-the-counter appetite stimulant
   b. Serve familiar and favorite foods
   c. Let them know that if the client does not eat, he might die
   d. Discuss this with the client's friends and family and see what they recommend doing

10. It is very important to follow safety guidelines when preparing food for the person with AIDS, because:

    a. Food-borne illnesses can cause death.

    b. You might become infected with HIV.

    c. You might infect family members with HIV.

    d. It is not important to follow safety guidelines regarding food preparation.

11. While preparing food for the person with AIDS, you should do all of the following EXCEPT:

    a. Wash your hands frequently.

    b. keep all utensils, counter tops, and cutting boards clean.

    c. Wash and cook foods thoroughly.

    d. Add lots of spicy seasonings to the food to make it taste better.

12. AIDS clients who have infections of the mouth and esophagus may need to eat food that is:

    a. Spicy

    b. Low in acid

    c. Dry

    d. Chewy

13. Someone who has nausea and vomiting should:

    a. Eat mostly dairy products

    b. Eat high-fat and spicy foods

    c. Drink liquids and eat salty foods

    d. Reduce liquid intake

14. The "BRAT" diet is helpful for:

    a. Diarrhea

    b. Weight gain

    c. Nausea and vomiting

    d. Headaches

15. Fluids are important for clients who have diarrhea because:

    a. Diarrhea rapidly depletes the body of fluids.

    b. Diarrhea can be prevented by drinking a lot of fluids.

    c. Diarrhea is an infection that can be flushed out by fluids.

    d. Diarrhea can make a client's throat dry.

16. The following is helpful in dealing with neuropathy:

    a. Pain medications

    b. Wearing tight shoes

    c. Using a bed cradle

    d. Tucking in bedsheets tightly

17. People with AIDS often suffer from anxiety and depression because:

    a. AIDS is curable.

    b. Others may have positive attitudes about people with AIDS.

    c. They may have already lost friends and family members to the disease.

    d. Their cognitive ability is not affected.

17. Describe normal changes of aging in the brain

Multiple Choice.

1. The ability to think logically and quickly is called:

    a. Cognition

    b. Dementia

    c. Awareness

    d. Respiration

2. Cognitive impairment affects:

    a. Social security reform

    b. Motor skills

    c. Concentration and memory

    d. Diet

3. Home health aides can help elderly clients by:

    a. Doing as much as possible for them

    b. Encouraging them to make lists of things to remember

    c. Reminding them every time they forget something

    d. Telling them to think as hard as they can

18. Discuss confusion and delirium

Short Answer.

1. What ten actions can you take when you are helping care for a client who is confused?

_____

_____

_____

_____

_____

_____

_____

_____

_____

2. Name four possible causes of delirium.

_____

_____

_____

_____

_____

19. Define dementia and recognize its causes

True or False.

1. _____ Dementia is the loss of mental abilities such as thinking, remembering, reasoning, and communicating.

2. _____ Dementia is a normal part of aging.

20. Describe Alzheimer's disease and identify its stages and related behaviors

True or False.

1. _____ Alzheimer's disease begins with forgetfulness and confusion and progresses to complete loss of all ability to care for oneself.

2. _____ Different people with Alzheimer's disease may show different symptoms at different times.

3. _____ A home health aide should perform as many activities as possible for clients with Alzheimer's disease.

4. _____ Alzheimer's disease cannot be cured.

21. Identify personal attitudes helpful in caring for people with AD or any dementia

Short Answer.

For each of the following personal attitudes in caring for Alzheimer's clients, briefly describe why each attitude is helpful.

1. Do not take it personally. Why?

_____

_____

_____

_____

_____

_____

2. Put yourself in their shoes. Why?

_____

_____

_____

_____

_____

_____

_____

3. Work with the symptoms and behaviors you see. Why?

_____

_____

_____

_____

_____

4. Work as a team. Why?

_____

_____

_____

_____

_____

5. Take care of yourself. Why?

_____

_____

_____

_____

_____

_____

6. Work with family members. Why?

_____

_____

_____

_____

_____

7. Remember the goals of the client care plan. Why?

_____

_____

_____

_____

_____

22. List strategies for better communication for clients with Alzheimer's disease

True or False.

1. _____ When communicating with an Alzheimer's client, speak in a calm, quiet manner.

2. _____ Plenty of noise and distractions can help the client cope with having Alzheimer's disease.

3. _____ Perseveration means to wander constantly.

4. _____ When working with an Alzheimer's client, you may have to repeat yourself several times.

5. _____ You should always use the same words and phrases when repeating something.

6. _____ A drawing of a toilet can be a form of communication.

7. _____ Nonverbal communication is not effective when dealing with Alzheimer's clients.

Multiple Choice.

8. When communicating with a client with AD, you should:

    a. Approach the client from behind.

    b. Stand as close as you are comfortable to the client.

    c. Communicate in a loud, busy place.

    d. Speak slowly, using a lower voice than normal.

9. If a client is frightened or anxious, which of the following should you NOT do?

    a. Check your body language so you do not appear tense or hurried.

    b. Turn the television or radio off.

    c. Use complex sentences.

    d. List self-care steps one at a time.

10. If a client perseverates, this mean he or she is:

    a. Repeating words, phrases, questions, or actions

    b. Suggesting words that sound correct

    c. Hallucinating

    d. Gesturing instead of speaking to you

11. If the client does not remember how to perform basic tasks, you should:

    a. Do everything for him or her.

    b. Encourage the client to do what he or she can.

    c. Skip explaining each activity.

    d. Say "don't" as often as you feel is necessary.

23. Describe a safe environment for a client with AD

Short Answer.

1. List three things you can do to organize the home for disoriented clients.

   _____

   _____

   _____

   _____

2. List three things you can do to organize the home for clients who wander.

   _____

   _____

   _____

   _____

3. List three things you can do to organize the home for clients who pace.

   _____

   _____

   _____

24. Explain general principles that will assist clients with personal care

Short Answer.

What three principles will help you give all clients the best care?

_____

_____

_____

_____

25. List and describe interventions for problems with common activities of daily living (ADLs)

Short Answer.

For each of the following statements, write "good idea" if the statement is a good idea for clients with Alzheimer's disease, and "bad idea" if the statement is a bad idea.

1. Use nonslip mats, tub seats, and hand holds to ensure safety during bathing.

   _____

2. Always bathe the client at the same time every day, even if he or she is agitated.

   _____

3. Always use the same steps and explain what you are doing the same way every time.

   _____

4. Do not attempt to groom the client, since he or she may not enjoy this.

   _____

5. Choose clothes that are simple to put on.

   _____

6. If the client is incontinent, do not give him or her fluids.

   _____

7. Mark the restroom with a sign as a reminder of when to use it and where it is.

   _____

8. Check the skin regularly for signs of irritation.

   _____

9. Follow Standard Precautions when caring for the client.

_____

10. Do not encourage exercise as this will make the client more agitated.

_____

11. Serve finger foods if the client tends to wander during meals.

_____

12. Schedule meals at the same time every day.

_____

13. Serve new kinds of foods as often as possible to stimulate the client.

_____

14. Offer one course at a time, using one utensil at a time.

_____

15. Monitor weight accurately and frequently.

_____

16. Do not encourage independence as this can lead to aggressive behavior.

_____

17. Provide a daily calendar to encourage activities.

_____

18. Reward positive behavior with smiles, hugs, warm touches, and thank-yous.

_____

26. List and describe interventions for common difficult behaviors related to Alzheimer's disease

Scenarios.

1. Mr. Imfeld is showing signs of agitation. Patrick, his caregiver, notices that the television in the next room is playing a very loud commercial. What should Patrick do?

_____

_____

_____

Mr. Imfeld still seems agitated. What can Patrick do now?

_____

_____

_____

_____

_____

2. Mrs. Drew is wandering around the house aimlessly. Her caregiver, Ruth, knows that she has just eaten and has gone to the restroom. Mrs. Drew had a long nap earlier. What can Ruth do about Mrs. Drew's wandering?

_____

_____

_____

_____

3. Mrs. Drew becomes extremely agitated when her new caregiver, Ruth, tries to give her a tub bath. Mrs. Drew's daughter is present and tells Ruth that her mother is used to taking showers. What can Ruth do?

_____

_____

_____

_____

4. Lately, Fran notices that Mr. Young seems withdrawn and listless (has no energy). He refuses to eat and seems to have lost all interest in his favorite activities. What can Fran do?

_____

_____

_____

_____

5. Mrs. Montoya persists in asking her caregiver, Jamie, who she is. What should Jamie do?

_____

_____

_____

_____

_____

27. Describe creative therapies for clients with AD

Fill in the Blank.

Fill in the blanks with the words listed below.

Activity therapy   Reminiscence therapy

Reality orientation   Validation therapy

1. Encouraging the client to talk about the past and explore memories is

_____.

2. Using calendars, clocks, signs, and lists to help the client remember who and where she is is called

_____.

3. Using activities to prevent boredom and frustration and improve self-esteem is

_____.

4. Letting the client believe he lives in the past or in imaginary circumstances, without attempting to reorient him is

_____.

28. Describe how Alzheimer's disease may affect the client's family

Short Answer.

1. Why might it be difficult for families of people who have AD?

_____

_____

_____

_____

_____

_____

2. What two major resources affect the ability of clients' families to cope with AD?

_____

_____

_____

_____

_____

_____

29. Identify community resources available to people with Alzheimer's disease and their families

Short Answer.

List four resources a person with AD and their families can turn to in times of need.

_____

_____

_____

_____

_____

_____

_____

21

Clean, Safe, and Healthy Environments

1. Describe how housekeeping affects physical and psychological well-being

Short Answer.

What are some reasons you should maintain an orderly and clean household for your client?

_____

_____

_____

_____

_____

_____

_____

_____

2. List qualities needed to manage a home and describe general housekeeping guidelines

True or False.

1. _____ Your primary responsibility as a home health aide is to clean your client's kitchen.

2. _____ You should expect that all members of the household will be able to help with housekeeping.

3. _____ Your assignment might include managing a client's finances.

4. _____ You may need to be flexible with regard to household maintenance.

5. _____ As a home health aide, you will never have to do a client's laundry.

6. _____ You will be solely responsible for determining which home maintenance activities you will perform.

7. _____ You should be sensitive towards your client's customs and beliefs.

8. _____ You need to use cleaning materials and methods that are acceptable to and approved by clients and their families.

9. _____ Using proper body mechanics is not important in performing housekeeping chores.

3. Describe cleaning products and equipment

True or False.

1. _____ All-purpose cleaners can be used on several types of surfaces.

2. _____ It is okay to mix bleach and ammonia to clean surfaces that are really stained.

3. _____ Abrasive cleaners are used mostly for bathing clients.

4. _____ A sponge is generally used to soften and remove soil on washable surfaces.

5. _____ Vacuum cleaner bags should be checked frequently.

6. _____ Some cleaning products can cause burns.

7. _____ You can use a specialty cleaner to clean the oven.

8. _____ There are five basic types of home cleaning products available.

4. Describe proper cleaning methods for living areas, kitchens, bathrooms, and storage areas

Multiple Choice.

1. Examples of essential items which should be kept close by the client include:

   a. Tissues

   b. Potato chips

   c. Nail polish

   d. Cosmetics

2. Frequent causes of falls and accidents in the home are:

   a. Well-lit hallways

   b. Wet floors

   c. Clean floors

   d. Leftover food scraps

3. In the kitchen, diseases may be transmitted by:

   a. Hot water

   b. Medications

   c. Contaminated food surfaces

   d. Bleach

4. It is a good idea to dust this often, unless the client has allergies:

   a. Five times a week

   b. Once a week

   c. Once every two months

   d. Twice a month

5. You can defrost a freezer quickly by:

   a. Using a warm knife to chip at the ice

   b. Lighting matches near the ice

   c. Using a blow torch

   d. Placing pans of hot water in it

6. In order to remove odors, you can use:

   a. Flour

   b. Baking soda

   c. Sugar

   d. Baking powder

7. You can sterilize dishes by:

   a. Using a dishwasher

   b. Using cold water

   c. Using an oven cleaner

   d. Drying them with a dish towel

8. How often should you dispose of garbage?

   a. Daily

   b. Weekly

   c. Monthly

   d. Bi-annually

9. Basic bathroom hygiene includes:

   a. Washing from dirty areas to clean areas

   b. Placing soiled towels on the bathroom sink

   c. Scrubbing the tub and shower after each use

   d. Leave toothbrushes in the sink

10. Instead of glass cleaner, you can mix water and:

    a. White wine

    b. White vinegar

    c. Apple juice

    d. Spray starch

11. In what situation do mold and mildew grow best?

    a. In extreme cold

    b. In dry heat

    c. When it is moist and warm

    d. In frigid winds

12. How many parts water should you dilute bleach with to clean bathroom surfaces?

    a. Twelve parts

    b. Four parts

    c. One part

    d. Six parts

13. Vacuum floors and rugs at least:

    a. Once a month

    b. Twice a week

    c. Once a week

    d. Once a day

5. Describe how to prepare a cleaning schedule

Create a sample cleaning schedule for an immobile client.

Immediately:

_____

_____

_____

_____

_____

Daily:

_____

_____

_____

_____

_____

Weekly:

_____

_____

_____

_____

_____

Monthly:

_____

_____

_____

_____

_____

Less often:

_____

_____

_____

_____

_____

6. List special housekeeping procedures to use when infection is present

Word Search.

Complete each of the following sentences and find your answers in the word search.

1. _____ any surfaces that contact body fluids, such as a _____, urinal, and toilet.

2. Frequently remove _____ containing used tissues.

3. Keep any _____ of urine or stool in double bags away from food.

4. Take special _____ in housecleaning when you know the client has a known infectious disease.

5. Use _____ dishes and utensils for the infected client.

6. Wash dishes in hot soapy water with _____, and rinse in _____ water.

7. _____ the client's bathroom daily

j	n	q	v	v	b	v	o	o	r	p	o	e	s
s	d	a	k	b	w	l	n	e	r	i	s	i	n
v	g	j	p	d	b	i	e	e	i	p	l	p	e
f	k	d	o	d	f	o	c	a	t	y	v	a	m
y	z	e	k	o	e	a	i	f	c	t	m	h	i
f	z	b	u	d	u	b	h	l	j	h	p	c	c
q	t	l	n	t	m	b	c	d	i	d	v	x	e
r	a	b	i	c	l	e	a	n	z	n	n	m	p
z	p	o	e	t	a	r	a	p	e	s	g	t	s
u	n	r	j	p	q	y	s	k	p	z	r	c	b
s	d	i	s	i	n	f	e	c	t	a	o	t	x
j	r	l	a	t	p	o	f	x	s	d	w	x	u
u	r	n	z	d	z	w	h	h	k	b	f	u	t
u	y	a	d	p	z	x	j	j	m	c	e	f	k

7. Explain how to do laundry and care for clothes

Crossword.

Across

4. Whites and towels should generally be washed in _____ water.

5. If clients can do their own mending, they may just need you to _____ a needle.

6. Liquid chlorine bleach removes stains and _____ clothing.

8. The safest temperature for most garments is _____.

10. There are three types of bleach: liquid chlorine, powdered chlorine, and _____ bleach.

11. A delicate fabric requires _____ time in the dryer.

12. Brightly colored fabrics should be washed in _____ water.

Down

1. Before washing is done, certain especially dirty or stained items should be _____.

2. Every time you use the dryer, you should clean the _____.

3. Delicate or fragile items should be washed on the _____ cycle.

6. Folding clothes immediately after they are dried reduces _____.

7. Pressing silks on the wrong side helps prevent them from becoming _____.

8. Bleach should always be diluted with _____.

9. Sturdy permanent press items and cottons can be washed on the _____ setting.

12. You should iron collars and _____ first.

8. List special laundry precautions to use when infection is present

True or False.

1. _____ When handling laundry for a client who has an infectious disease, use cold water.

2. _____ You should wear gloves when doing an infectious client's laundry.

3. _____ If an infectious disease is present, do not use liquid bleach.

4. _____ Keep an infectious client's laundry separate from other family members' laundry.

5. _____ Sort an infectious client's laundry and put in plastic bags.

6. _____ Use a disinfectant in all loads.

9. List guidelines for teaching housekeeping skills to clients' family members

Scenario.

Read the following scenario and decide how to respond.

Dave, a home health aide, is explaining to Mrs. Crawford's family how to protect against infectious diseases when doing the laundry and cleaning the kitchen. He has written a long list of instructions, and when he is done explaining, two family members still seem confused about some key points. How should Dave respond in this situation?

_____

_____

_____

_____

_____

_____

_____

_____

_____

_____

_____

_____

_____

_____

10. Discuss the importance of sleep and explain why careful bedmaking is important

Short Answer.

List three reasons why careful bedmaking is important.

_____

_____

_____

_____

_____

11. Identify hazardous household materials

Short Answer.

Identify five hazardous household materials.

_____

_____

_____

_____

_____

_____

22

Clients' Nutritional Needs

1. Describe the importance of good nutrition and list the six basic nutrients

Short Answer.

Read the following sentences and mark which of the six basic nutrients it is describing. Use a "P" for proteins, "C" for carbohydrates, "F" for fats, "V" for vitamins, "M" for minerals, and "W" for water.

1. _____ Good sources of these are fish, meat, dried beans, and cheese.

2. _____ Without this, a person can only live a few days.

3. _____ These help the body store energy.

4. _____ These add flavor to food and help to absorb certain vitamins.

5. _____ Beans and rice are examples of complementary _____.

6. _____ Examples of these are butter, oil, and salad dressing.

7. _____ They are essential for tissue growth and repair.

8. _____ The body cannot produce most of these.

9. _____ These provide fiber.

10. _____ Examples of these include bread, cereal, and potatoes.

11. _____ This is the most essential nutrient for life.

12. _____ These can be classified as monounsaturated, polyunsaturated, and saturated.

13. _____ Through perspiration, this helps to maintain body temperature.

14. _____ These can be fat-soluble or water-soluble.

15. _____ One-half to two-thirds of our body weight is this.

16. _____ Iron and calcium are examples of these.

2. Describe the USDA's MyPyramid

Labeling.

Looking at the USDA's MyPyramid below, fill in the seven areas.

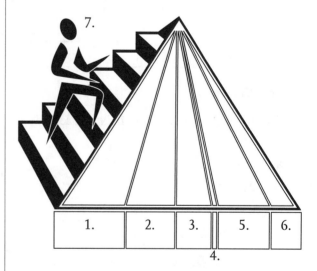

1. _____

2. _____

3. _____

4. _____

5. _____

6. _____

7. _____

Name: _____

Short Answer.

8. Describe your diet during the last 24 hours and break it down into food groups and servings.

_____

_____

_____

_____

_____

_____

_____

_____

_____

_____

_____

_____

Multiple Choice.

9. The Pyramid is made up of six colored bands, which represent:
   a. Grains
   b. Different food groups
   c. Meat and beans
   d. Ideal weights

10. What types of food should form the "base" of a healthy diet?
    a. Foods that are nutrient-dense and low in fat
    b. Foods that are high in fat and sugar
    c. Meats and dairy products
    d. Oils containing fatty acids

11. Most of your fruit choices should be:
    a. Frozen fruit
    b. Smoothies
    c. Cut-up fruit
    d. Fruit juice

12. How much vigorous activity does the USDA recommend you get per day?
    a. 60 minutes
    b. 20 minutes
    c. 10 minutes
    d. 30 minutes

13. Wheat, rice, oats, cornmeal, and barley are examples of which food group?
    a. Vegetables
    b. Fruits
    c. Grains
    d. Meat and beans

3. Identify ways to assist clients in maintaining fluid balance

True or False.

1. _____ Drinking 12 ounces of water per day is the recommended amount for most people.

2. _____ Fluid overload occurs when the body is unable to handle the amount of fluid consumed.

3. _____ The sense of thirst diminishes in elderly people.

4. _____ People can become dehydrated by vomiting too much.

5. _____ A symptom of fluid overload is flushed, dry skin.

6. _____ In order to prevent dehydration, you should encourage clients to drink every time you see them.

7. _____ A symptom of dehydration is dark urine.

4. Identify nutritional problems of the elderly or ill

Short Answer.

1. What can unintended weight loss lead to?

_____

_____

_____

_____

_____

_____

_____

2. List five things to observe and report to your supervisor about unintended weight loss.

_____

_____

_____

_____

_____

_____

_____

Word Search.

Complete each of the following sentences and find your answers in the word search.

3. Encourage clients to
   _____.

4. Provide _____
   before and after meals.

5. Honor _____
   likes and dislikes.

6. Offer many different kinds of foods and
   _____.

7. Allow enough _____ to
   finish eating.

8. Notify your supervisor if a client has trouble
   using _____.

9. Position clients sitting
   _____ for feeding.

10. If client has had a loss of
    _____, ask
    about it.

11. Record meal/snack
    _____.

e	u	a	x	w	e	r	a	c	l	a	r	o	u
e	k	j	i	l	n	s	t	u	m	b	b	p	s
j	e	a	e	j	e	t	s	w	y	e	r	y	e
l	r	t	t	p	s	f	l	v	v	i	g	z	c
q	c	x	i	n	z	k	n	e	g	p	a	p	d
l	j	o	f	t	i	g	r	h	p	y	e	p	o
i	v	p	i	c	e	a	t	u	e	s	v	b	h
b	w	m	v	m	g	p	c	m	d	v	a	a	x
j	n	o	u	e	j	z	p	l	u	j	q	l	m
d	o	q	s	w	f	z	l	a	o	b	w	m	w
t	a	t	d	b	n	t	o	x	m	e	c	l	p
c	a	o	o	u	d	x	g	e	k	d	m	z	n
e	o	w	i	x	v	a	g	c	c	d	c	i	u
f	u	t	e	n	s	i	l	s	i	i	w	c	t

Short Answer.

12. What is a nasogastric tube?

_____

_____

_____

_____

_____

_____

13. What is a gastrostomy?

_____

_____

_____

_____

_____

14. What is total parenteral nutrition (TPN)?

_____

_____

_____

_____

_____

_____

_____

5. Demonstrate awareness of regional, cultural, and religious food preferences

Short Answer.

Briefly describe some of the foods you ate while growing up. Were there any special dishes that your family made that were related to your culture, religion, or region?

_____

_____

_____

_____

_____

_____

_____

_____

_____

_____

_____

_____

6. List and define common health claims on food labels

Fill in the Blank.

1. _____ meat, poultry, eggs, and dairy products come from animals that are given no antibiotics or growth hormones.

2. _____ products may contain artificial sweeteners, such as saccharin or aspartame.

3. If a product is labeled _____ or _____, it usually does not contain much fat.

4. The claims of _____, "healthy," or "good for you" may have little or no meaning.

5. Clients who must reduce their sodium or salt intake should eat foods labeled _____ or _____.

6. The best way to limit _____ is to avoid foods containing animal fats.

7. Explain the information on the FDA-required Nutrition Facts label

Multiple Choice.

1. Total calories from fat should be no more than:
   a. 30%
   b. 50%
   c. 10%
   d. 2%

2. If the percentage of daily totals for vitamins and minerals exceeds 50%, you know that:
   a. It might make you sick.
   b. It is more than you need for the day.
   c. It is a good source of that vitamin or mineral.
   d. It should only be consumed in intervals.

3. For which of the following does the FDA-required label NOT give amounts?
   a. Herbs
   b. Sodium
   c. Calories
   d. Serving size

4. The standardized nutrition label on all packaged foods is called:
   a. The label
   b. Food information
   c. Nutrition facts
   d. Serving size information

5. The recommended daily totals are based on a _____ calorie diet.
   a. 2,500
   b. 2,000
   c. 1,000
   d. 5,000

8. Explain special diets

Matching.

Read the following sentences and identify what special diet each is describing. Choose from the diets listed below.

a. Low-Sodium Diet

b. Fluid-Restricted Diet

c. Low-Protein Diet

d. Low-Fat/Low-Cholesterol Diet

e. Modified Calorie Diet

f. Bland Diet

g. Dietary Management of Diabetes

h. Soft Diet and Mechanical Soft Diet

i. Pureed Diet

1. _____ To prevent further heart or kidney damage, physicians may restrict a client's fluid intake.

2. _____ This diet consists of soft or chopped foods that are easy to chew and swallow, and is ordered for clients who have trouble chewing and swallowing due to dental problems or other medical conditions.

3. _____ In addition to restricted intake of fluids and sodium, people who have kidney disease may also be on this diet.

4. _____ People at risk for heart attacks and heart disease may be placed on these. This diet includes limiting fatty meats, egg yolks, and fried foods.

5. _____ Calories and carbohydrates must be carefully regulated in this diet. The types of foods and the amounts are determined by the person's nutritional and energy requirements.

6. _____ Salt is restricted in this diet. Other high-sodium foods, such as ham, nuts, pickles, and canned soups, will be limited.

7. _____ Used for losing weight or preventing additional weight gain.

8. _____ This diet of food has been blended or ground into a thick paste of baby-food consistency is often used for people who have trouble chewing and/or swallowing more textured foods.

9. _____ This diet avoids foods that produce or increase levels of acid in the stomach, such as alcohol, and beverages containing caffeine.

Short Answer.

Read the following meals and modify to fit the specific special diets.

10. **Regular diet**
    BREAKFAST
    Scrambled eggs
    Bacon
    Toast with butter
    Whole milk

    Low fat/cholesterol diet
    BREAKFAST

    _____

    _____

    _____

    _____

    _____

    _____

11. **Regular diet**
    LUNCH
    Ham sandwich
    Potato chips
    Canned soup
    Cookies

    Low sodium diet
    LUNCH

    _____

    _____

    _____

    _____

    _____

Name:_____

12. **Regular diet**
DINNER
Steak
Baked potato with sour cream
Sauteed green beans
Chocolate cream pie

Low fat/cholesterol diet
DINNER

_____

_____

_____

_____

_____

_____

23

Meal Planning, Shopping, Preparation, and Storage

1. Explain how to prepare a basic food plan and list food shopping guidelines

Short Answer.

Make a basic food plan for Monday through Friday. Include breakfast, lunch, dinner, and snacks.

MONDAY

Breakfast

Snack

Lunch

Snack

Dinner

Snack

TUESDAY

Breakfast

Snack

Lunch

Snack

Dinner

Snack

WEDNESDAY

Breakfast

Snack

Lunch

Snack

Dinner

Snack

THURSDAY

Breakfast

Snack

Lunch

Snack

Dinner

Snack

FRIDAY

Breakfast

Snack

Lunch

Snack

Dinner

Snack

Name:_____

Fill in the Blank.

1. Avoid _____ or ready-made foods because they are more expensive.

2. If you have the time, make food from scratch and buy _____ items.

3. Read _____ for ingredients that may be harmful to your client.

4. Estimate the _____ by dividing the total cost by the number of servings.

5. For clients on a low-fat diet, take the _____ off chicken and turkey parts.

6. Buy fresh foods that are in season when they are at their _____ flavor.

7. Large amounts or larger sizes are usually more _____.

8. Cheaper cuts of meat tend to have more _____ in bones and fat.

Short Answer.

9. List four factors to consider when buying food.

_____

_____

_____

_____

_____

2. List guidelines for safe food preparation

True or False.

1. _____ You should wash your hands before, but not after, handling food.

2. _____ Sponges can be washed in the dishwasher to disinfect them.

3. _____ Defrost frozen foods on the countertops.

4. _____ Food can be left out safely for five hours.

5. _____ You need to cook poultry thoroughly to kill microorganisms.

6. _____ Food-borne illnesses affect up to one million people each year.

7. _____ It is best to use plastic cutting boards for raw meat.

8. _____ It is not necessary to change knives between cutting fresh meat and vegetables.

9. _____ It is especially important to prepare food safely for people who have weakened immune systems.

10. _____ Elderly people are at increased risk for a food-borne illness because often they cannot taste if food is spoiled.

3. Identify methods of food preparation

Fill in the Blank.

Read the following descriptions and identify what method of food preparation it is. The methods are listed below. Some methods will be used more than once.

baking	microwaving
boiling	poaching
braising	roasting
broiling	sauteing
frying	steaming

1. _____ Safe for defrosting, reheating, and cooking, but this method can cause "cold spots."

2. _____ Cooked in barely boiling water or other liquids, this is an ideal way to prepare fish and eggs.

3. _____ Used mostly for meats and poultry, this method requires basting.

4. _____ This is a healthy way to prepare vegetables.

5. _____ Used mostly for meats, it involves cooking food close to the source of heat at a high temperature for a short time.

6. _____ The best method for cooking pasta, noodles, and rice.

7. _____ Done in a moderate oven, this method is used for many foods such as breads, fish, and vegetables.

8. _____ A quick way to cook vegetables and meats by using a small amount of oil in a frying pan and stirring constantly.

9. _____ A small amount of water is boiled in the bottom of a saucepan and food is set over it on a rack.

10. _____ The least healthy way to cook, this method uses a lot of fat.

11. _____ You can use this method to melt cheese or brown the top of a casserole.

12. _____ A slow-cooking method that uses moist heat to cook meat or vegetables at a temperature just below boiling.

4. Identify four methods of low-fat food preparation

Fill in the Blank.

1. _____ allows fats in meat to drip out before food is consumed, which lowers fat content.

2. Plan meals around _____, which are the base of the food pyramid.

3. Sometimes high-fat ingredients can be _____ to lower the fat content of a recipe.

4. _____ meat on paper towels after you brown it.

5. Leave out _____ on sandwiches or on top of casseroles.

6. An example of a low-fat meal based on grains is beans and _____.

7. Boiling, steaming, broiling, and _____ are all methods of cooking that require little fat.

8. Try substituting _____ for mayonnaise or sour cream.

5. List four guidelines for safe food storage

Multiple Choice.

1. After shopping, which foods should be put away first?
   a. Crackers
   b. Dairy
   c. Grains
   d. Cereals

2. It is a good idea to keep easily-spoiled items in the:
   a. Door of the refrigerator
   b. Cupboard
   c. Rear of the refrigerator
   d. Pantry

3. Refrigerator temperature should be at:
   a. 0°F
   b. 36°F - 40°F
   c. 10°F - 20°F
   d. 62°F - 66°F

4. You can safely leave foods out for _____ hours.
   a. Five
   b. Three
   c. Two
   d. Twelve

5. If you are not sure whether food is spoiled, you should:

    a. Discard it.

    b. Serve it and see if anyone complains or feels ill.

    c. Cook it for a longer time than usual.

    d. Smell it after cooking it to be sure it is okay.

6. Describe guidelines for assisting with eating

Multiple Choice.

1. When assisting clients with eating, encourage them to do whatever they can for themselves. This does NOT include:

    a. If a client can hold a napkin, she should.

    b. If a client can use special adaptive utensils, she should.

    c. If a client can hold and eat finger foods, she should.

    d. Making the food choices for the client, rather than letting her choose

2. Ways to promote a client's dignity while feeding include:

    a. Telling him, "Hurry up. I've still got to give you a bath."

    b. Asking him, "What would you like to try first?"

    c. Looking around the room while he is eating

    d. Mixing food whether or not the client has requested it

True or False.

3. _____ Clients who must be fed are often embarrassed and depressed about their dependence on another person.

4. _____ Alternate food and drink while feeding.

5. _____ Sit higher than a client while feeding.

6. _____ You should give a client your full attention during eating.

7. _____ When feeding a client, make sure the client's mouth is empty before giving another bite of food or sip of beverage.

8. _____ A client should be fed lying flat on his back.

Short Answer.

9. In a few words, describe how you might feel if you needed help to perform activities of daily living (ADLs), such as eating or bathing.

    _____

    _____

    _____

    _____

    _____

    _____

    _____

    _____

    _____

    _____

    _____

    _____

7. Describe eating and swallowing problems a client may have

Short Answer.

1. List five ways to prevent aspiration.

    _____

    _____

    _____

    _____

    _____

    _____

    _____

    _____

    _____

_____

_____

_____

_____

2. List seven signs and symptoms of a swallowing problem, or dysphagia.

_____

_____

_____

_____

_____

_____

_____

_____

3. List the three basic thickened consistencies that clients may be restricted to consuming, and describe each.

_____

_____

_____

_____

_____

_____

_____

_____

24

Managing Time, Energy, and Money

1. Explain three ways to work more efficiently

Short Answer.

1. For each of the three ways of working more efficiently described in this learning objective, give an example (other than what it is in the book) of how you can put the method into action.

_____

_____

_____

_____

_____

_____

_____

_____

_____

_____

_____

_____

_____

2. List five ways to conserve time and energy.

_____

_____

_____

_____

_____

2. Describe how to follow an established work plan with the client and family

Short Answer.

Pick the busiest day you will have next week, and draft a work plan for that day. List tasks to complete and prioritize them.

_____

_____

_____

_____

_____

_____

_____

_____

_____

_____

_____

3. Discuss ways to handle inappropriate requests

Scenario.

Read the following scenario and answer the question.

Richard, a home health aide, is preparing to leave his client's home for the day. Mr. Perez, his client, demands that Richard buy him some soup at the grocery store before he leaves. This errand is not in the care plan, but Mr. Perez tells him that he really wants some soup. Mr. Perez begins to cry. What should Richard do in this situation?

Name: _____

_____

_____

_____

True or False.

2. _____ It is fine to use your client's money for your own things as long as you pay it back.

3. _____ Use cash whenever possible.

4. _____ It is a good idea to estimate the amount of money you will need before you request it.

5. _____ Return receipts to client or family member as soon as possible.

6. _____ It is a good idea to keep a record of the money you have spent and where you have spent it.

7. _____ You are not responsible for lost money.

8. _____ Keep a client's cash separate from yours.

9. _____ If a client is unsure about his budget, you should give him advice about how much money to spend and where to spend it.

4. List five money-saving homemaking tips

Short Answer.

List and briefly explain the five money-saving tips.

_____

_____

_____

_____

_____

_____

_____

_____

5. List guidelines for handling a client's money

Short Answer.

1. What are your state's guidelines for handling a client's money?

_____

_____

_____

_____

25

Caring for Yourself and Your Career

1. Explain how to conduct a job search

Short Answer.

List three resources you should try when looking for potential employers.

_____

_____

_____

_____

_____

_____

_____

_____

_____

2. Identify documents that may be required when applying for a job

Short Answer.

List four documents that you may need when you apply for a job.

_____

_____

_____

_____

_____

_____

_____

_____

_____

3. Demonstrate completing an effective job application

Short Answer.

Complete the sample job application.

Employment Application

Personal Information

Name:	Date:

Social Security Number:

Home Address:

City, State, Zip:

Home Phone:	Business Phone:

US Citizen?	If Not, Give Visa No. and Expiration Date:

Position Applying For

Title:	Salary Desired:
Referred By:	Date Available:

Education

High School (Name, City, State):

Graduation Date:

Technical or Undergraduate School:

Dates Attended:	Degree Major:

References

Name: _____

4. Demonstrate competence in job interview techniques

Short Answer.

Write "Yes" or "No" next to the descriptions below to indicate whether or not it is appropriate for a job interview.

1. _____ Arrive a couple of minutes late for the interview

2. _____ Look happy to be there

3. _____ Ask, "Do you mind if I smoke?"

4. _____ Wear very little jewelry

5. _____ Ask, "How many hours would I work?"

6. _____ Bring child with her since she could not find a babysitter

7. _____ Say, "I won't work with patients with AIDS."

8. _____ Sit up straight

9. _____ Ask, "What benefits do I receive with this job?"

10. _____ Shake hands with interviewer

11. _____ Eat a granola bar during the interview

12. _____ Ask, "Did I get the job?"

5. Discuss appropriate responses to criticism

Short Answer.

Read the following and mark whether they are examples of hostile or constructive criticism. Use an "H" for hostile and a "C" for constructive.

1. _____ "You are a horrible person."

2. _____ "If you weren't so slow, things might get done around here."

3. _____ "Some of your reports are not completed; try to be more accurate."

4. _____ "That was the worst meal I've ever eaten!"

5. _____ "I'm not sure that you understood what I meant. Let me rephrase the issue."

6. _____ "Where did you learn how to clean?"

7. _____ "That was a stupid idea."

8. _____ "That procedure could have been performed in a more efficient way."

9. _____ "Try to make more of an effort to listen carefully."

10. _____ "Stop being so lazy."

6. Identify effective ways to make a complaint to an employer or supervisor

Scenario.

Read the following scenario and answer the question.

Anne is a home health aide who works three days a week for her client, Mrs. Singer. Generally, Mrs. Singer's son, Wayne, is there as well, and he and Anne work as a team. Wayne finds a new job and cannot be home during the day anymore. The next time Anne arrives, Mrs. Singer is moody and distant. She is reluctant to follow the care plan and she tells Anne that she will not take a bath until Wayne comes home. She also refuses to eat food that Anne has cooked, insisting she can only eat her son's cooking. After some gentle urging, Anne gets Mrs. Singer to eat and take a bath.

The next time Anne works, Mrs. Singer drops her plate on the floor and tells Anne that she is a lousy cook. She tells her to fix a new meal and clean up the mess. Anne does both, although she feels very upset.

Should this be reported to a supervisor? If so, how?

_____

_____

_____

_____

_____

_____
_____
_____
_____
_____
_____

7. Identify guidelines for making job changes

Fill in the Blank.

1. You should always give your employer _____ weeks written notice that you will be leaving.

2. Potential future employers may talk with your past _____.

3. If you decide to change jobs, be _____.

8. List your state's requirements for maintaining certification

Short Answer.

1. How many hours of in-service education are required each year by your state?

_____
_____

2. How long is an absence from working allowed, without retraining, by your state?

_____
_____
_____

9. Describe continuing education for home health aides

True or False.

1. _____ The federal government requires 20 hours of continuing education each year.

2. _____ Treatments or regulations can change.

3. _____ States require less continuing education than the federal government.

4. _____ In-service continuing education courses help you keep your knowledge fresh.

Short Answer.

5. List three of the responsibilities a home health aide has for receiving continuing education.

_____
_____
_____
_____
_____
_____
_____
_____

10. Define stress and stressors, and list examples

Short Answer.

What are some things that make you experience stress? How do you react when you are stressed?

_____
_____
_____
_____
_____
_____
_____
_____
_____
_____

11. Explain ways to manage stress

Multiple Choice.

1. Stress is a(n) _____ response.

    a. Relaxation

    b. Physical and emotional

    c. rare

    d. supervisory

2. When your heart beats fast in stressful situations, it can be a result of the increase of the hormone

    a. Testosterone

    b. Estrogen

    c. Adrenaline

    d. Progesterone

3. Which of the following is NOT a physical result of the effects of stress?

    a. Increase in heart rate

    b. Increase in relaxation

    c. Increase in respiratory rate

    d. Increase in nervous system response

4. A healthy lifestyle is the result of:

    a. Eating when you are not hungry

    b. Exercising regularly

    c. Smoking a few cigarettes a week

    d. Complaining about your job

5. Which of the following is a sign that you are not managing stress?

    a. Preparing meals ahead of time

    b. Not being able to focus on your work

    c. Feeling alert and positive

    d. Taking deep breaths and relaxing

Short Answer.

6. List four places and/or people to whom you can turn to help you manage stress.

    _____

    _____

    _____

12. Demonstrate two effective relaxation techniques

Fill in the Blank.

1. When doing the body scan exercise, pay attention to breathing and

    _____.

2. A _____ exercise can help you feel refreshed in a short time.

3. When performing the waterfall exercise, breathe deeply and imagine the force of the water is washing away your

    _____.

4. Start at the balls of your

    _____ when doing the body scan relaxation exercise.

13. Describe how to develop a personal stress management plan

Short Answer.

Write out your own personal stress management plan. Be sure to include things like diet, exercise, relaxation exercise, entertainment, etc.

_____

_____

_____

_____

_____

_____

_____

_____

_____

_____

_____

_____

_____

_____

_____

_____

14. List five guidelines for managing time

Short Answer.

List five guidelines for managing time.

_____

_____

_____

_____

_____

15. Demonstrate an understanding of the basics of money management

Crossword.

Across

1. When you apply for a mortgage or car loan, the bank or lender will check your

   _____.

2. To control expenses, try writing down what you _____ each day.

4. Very few people _____ their money well.

6. Making a personal or household

   _____

   helps you start solving money problems.

Down

1. The interest charged on _____ _____ debt is often the highest interest charged on any loan.

2. _____ some amount every time you get a check. Ten percent is a good goal.

3. Reduce or avoid _____, such as to banks, mortgage companies, or credit card companies.

5. Set a cash _____ for the week and stick to it.

16. Demonstrate an understanding that money matters are emotional

Short Answer.

When was the last time you wanted something you could not afford? How did it make you feel? What did you do?

_____

_____

_____

_____

_____

_____

_____

_____

_____

_____

_____

_____

_____

17. List ways to remind yourself that your work is important, valuable, and meaningful

Short Answer.

What made you choose to be a home health aide?

_____

_____

_____

_____

_____

_____

_____

_____

_____

Procedure Checklists

5

Infection Control and Standard Precautions

Washing hands

✓ **Procedure Steps**

❑ 1. Turns on water at sink.

❑ 2. Angles arms down holding hands lower than elbows. Wets hands and wrists thoroughly.

❑ 3. Applies soap to hands.

❑ 4. Lathers all surfaces of hands, wrists, and fingers, producing friction, for at least 20 seconds.

❑ 5. Cleans nails by rubbing them in palm of other hand.

❑ 6. Rinses all surfaces of wrists, hands, and fingers, keeping hands lower than the elbows and the fingertips down.

❑ 7. Uses clean, dry paper towel to dry all surfaces of hands, wrists, and fingers.

❑ 8. Uses clean, dry paper towel or knee to turn off faucet, without contaminating hands.

❑ 9. Disposes of used paper towel(s) in wastebasket immediately after shutting off faucet.

Comments:

Putting on gloves

✓ **Procedure Steps**

❑ 1. Washes hands.

❑ 2. If right-handed, slides one glove on left hand (reverse, if left-handed).

❑ 3. With gloved hand takes second glove and slides other hand into the glove.

❑ 4. Interlaces fingers to smooth out folds and create a comfortable fit.

❑ 5. Carefully looks for tears, holes, or spots. Replaces the glove if necessary.

❑ 6. If wearing a gown, pulls the cuff of the gloves over the sleeve of gown.

Comments:

Taking off gloves

✓ **Procedure Steps**

❑ 1. Touches only the outside of one glove and pulls the first glove off, turning it inside out.

❑ 2. With ungloved hand, reaches two fingers inside the remaining glove. Does not touch any part of the outside.

❑ 3. Pulls down, turning this glove inside out and over the first glove.

❑ 4. Disposes of gloves properly.

❑ 5. Washes hands.

Comments:

Putting on a gown

✓ **Procedure Steps**

❑ 1. Washes hands.

❑ 2. Opens gown without shaking it. Slips arms into the sleeves and pulls gown on.

❏ 3. Ties neck ties.

❏ 4. Pulls gown until it completely covers clothing. Ties the back ties.

Comments:

Putting on mask and goggles

✓ **Procedure Steps**

❏ 1. Washes hands.

❏ 2. Picks up mask by top strings or elastic strap. Does not touch mask where it touches face.

❏ 3. Adjusts mask over nose and mouth. Ties top strings first, then bottom strings.

❏ 4. Puts on goggles.

Comments:

Disinfecting using wet heat

✓ **Procedure Steps**

❏ 1. Washes hands.

❏ 2. Places items in the pot and fills it with water, covering all items.

❏ 3. Places lid on pot and places pot on stove.

❏ 4. Turns on heat and brings water to a boil. Boils for 20 minutes.

❏ 5. Turns off heat. Allows items and water to cool.

❏ 6. After items have cooled, removes cover and then items. Places items on rack or towel to dry.

❏ 7. Washes and dries equipment. Returns to proper storage.

❏ 8. Washes hands.

❏ 9. Documents procedure.

Comments:

Disinfecting using dry heat

✓ **Procedure Steps**

❏ 1. Washes hands.

❏ 2. Places items in the pan and places pan or sheet in oven.

❏ 3. Turns on oven to 350° F and bakes for one hour.

❏ 4. Turns off heat. Allow items to cool.

❏ 5. After items have cooled, removes items.

❏ 6. Stores items.

❏ 7. Washes and dries equipment. Returns to proper storage.

❏ 8. Washes hands.

❏ 9. Documents procedure.

Comments:

7

Emergency Care and Disaster Preparation

Abdominal thrusts for the conscious person

✓ **Procedure Steps**

❏ 1. Stands behind person and brings arms under person's arms. Wraps arms around person's waist.

❑ 2. Makes a fist with one hand. Places flat, thumb side of the fist against person's abdomen, above the navel but below the breastbone.

❑ 3. Grasps the fist with other hand. Pulls both hands toward self and up, quickly and forcefully.

❑ 4. Repeats until object is pushed out or person loses consciousness.

❑ 5. Reports and documents incident.

Comments:

Clearing an obstructed airway in a conscious infant

✓ Procedure Steps

❑ 1. Lies the infant face down on forearm; if sitting, rests the arm holding the infant's torso on lap or thigh. Supports infant's jaw and head with your hand.

❑ 2. Delivers up to 5 back blows.

❑ 3. If the obstruction is not expelled, turns infant onto his back while supporting the head. Delivers up to 5 chest thrusts

❑ 4. Repeats, alternating 5 back blows and 5 chest compressions until object is pushed out or the infant loses consciousness.

❑ 5. Reports and documents incident.

Comments:

Responding to shock

✓ Procedure Steps

❑ 1. Has the person lie down on her back unless bleeding from the mouth or vomiting.

❑ 2. Controls bleeding if bleeding occurs.

❑ 3. Checks pulse and respirations if possible.

❑ 4. Keeps person as calm and comfortable as possible.

❑ 5. Maintains normal body temperature.

❑ 6. Elevates the feet unless person has a head or abdominal injury, breathing difficulties, or a fractured bone or back.

❑ 7. Does not give person anything to eat or drink.

❑ 8. Calls for help immediately.

❑ 9. Reports and documents incident.

Comments:

Responding to a heart attack

✓ Procedure Steps

❑ 1. Calls or has someone call emergency services. Calls supervisor.

❑ 2. Places person in a comfortable position. Encourages him to rest, and reassures him that he will not be left alone.

❑ 3. Loosens clothing around the neck.

❑ 4. Does not give person liquids or food.

❑ 5. If person takes heart medication, such as nitroglycerin, finds medication and offers it to him. Does not place medication in person's mouth.

❑ 6. Monitors person's breathing and pulse. If breathing stops or person has no pulse, performs CPR if trained to do so.

❑ 7. Stays with person until help arrives.

❑ 8. Reports and documents incident.

Comments:

Controlling bleeding

✓ **Procedure Steps**

☐ 1. Puts on gloves.

☐ 2. Holds thick sterile pad, clean pad, or a clean cloth against the wound.

☐ 3. Presses down hard directly on the bleeding wound until help arrives. Does not decrease pressure. Puts additional pads over the first pad if blood seeps through. Does not remove the first pad.

☐ 4. Raises the wound above the heart to slow down the bleeding.

☐ 5. When bleeding is under control, secures the dressing to keep it in place. Checks person for symptoms of shock. Stays with person until help arrives.

☐ 6. Removes gloves and washes hands.

☐ 7. Reports and documents incident.

Comments:

Responding to poisoning

✓ **Procedure Steps**

☐ 1. Looks for a container that will help determine what the client has taken or eaten. Using gloves, checks the mouth for chemical burns and notes breath odor.

☐ 2. Calls the local or state poison control center immediately. Follows instructions.

☐ 3. Notifies supervisor.

☐ 4. Reports and documents incident.

Comments:

Treating burns

✓ **Procedure Steps**

Minor burns:

☐ 1. Uses cool, clean water (not ice) to decrease the skin temperature and prevent further injury (does not use ointment, salve, or grease).

☐ 2. Dampens a clean cloth and covers burn.

☐ 3. Covers area with a dry, sterile gauze.

Serious burns:

☐ 1. Removes person from the source of burn.

☐ 2. Calls for emergency help.

☐ 3. Checks for breathing, pulse, and severe bleeding. Does not apply water.

☐ 4. Does not remove clothing from burned areas. Covers burn with thick, dry, sterile gauze or a clean cloth (does not apply water or use ointment, salve, or grease).

☐ 5. Elevates affected part after person lies down.

☐ 6. If the burn is covers a larger area, wraps person in a dry, clean sheet. Takes care not to rub the skin.

☐ 7. Waits for emergency medical help.

☐ 8. Reports and documents incident.

Comments:

Responding to seizures

✓ **Procedure Steps**

☐ 1. Lowers person to the floor.

☐ 2. Has someone call emergency services immediately. Does not leave person unless has to get medical help.

3. Moves furniture away to prevent injury. If a pillow is nearby, places it under his head.

4. Does not try to restrain the person.

5. Does not force anything between the person's teeth. Does not place hands in person's mouth.

6. Does not give liquids or food.

7. When the seizure is over, checks breathing.

8. Reports and documents incident.

Comments:

Responding to fainting

✓ Procedure Steps

1. Has person lie down or sit down before fainting occurs.

2. If person is in sitting position, has her bend forward and place her head between her knees. If person is lying flat on her back, elevates the legs.

3. Loosens any tight clothing.

4. Has person stay in position for at least five minutes after symptoms disappear.

5. Helps person get up slowly. Continues to observe him for symptoms of fainting.

6. Reports and documents incident.

Comments:

Responding to a nosebleed

✓ Procedure Steps

1. Elevates head of the bed or tells client to remain in sitting position. Offers tissues or a clean cloth.

2. Puts on gloves. Applies firm pressure over the bridge of the nose. Squeezes bridge of nose with thumb and forefinger.

3. Applies pressure consistently until bleeding stops.

4. Uses a cool cloth or ice wrapped in a cloth on back of neck, forehead, or upper lip to slow blood flow.

5. Reports and documents incident.

Comments:

Helping a client who has fallen

✓ Procedure Steps

1. Assesses client's condition and gets help if condition warrants it.

2. Looks for broken bones.

3. Asks client to move each body part separately to observe.

If sprain or fracture is suspected:

4. Calls supervisor and reports fall.

5. Keeps injured area in one position. Does not move client.

6. Keeps client covered with blanket.

If no injury is suspected:

4. Makes the client comfortable.

5. Calls supervisor and reports fall.

6. Does not move client until talked with supervisor.

Comments:

12

Transfers, Ambulation, and Positioning

Helping a client sit up using the arm lock

✓ **Procedure Steps**

☐ 1. Washes hands.

☐ 2. Explains procedure to client, speaking clearly, slowly, and directly. Maintains face-to-face contact whenever possible.

☐ 3. Provides privacy.

☐ 4. Adjusts the bed to safe working level, if possible. Locks bed wheels.

☐ 5. Stands facing the bed with legs about 12 inches apart and knees bent. Puts foot further from the bed slightly ahead of the other foot.

☐ 6. Places arm under client's armpit and grasps client shoulder, while client grasps caregiver's shoulder.

☐ 7. Reaches under client's head and places other hand on client's far shoulder. Has client bend knees. Bends own knees.

☐ 8. Rocks backward at the count of three and pulls client to sitting position.

☐ 9. Observes client for dizziness or weakness.

☐ 10. Returns bed to lowest position if raised.

☐ 11. Washes hands.

☐ 12. Documents procedure and any observations.

Comments:

Moving a client up in bed

✓ **Procedure Steps**

If client can assist:

☐ 1. Washes hands.

☐ 2. Explains procedure to client, speaking clearly, slowly, and directly. Maintains face-to-face contact whenever possible.

☐ 3. Provides privacy.

☐ 4. Adjusts the bed to safe working level, if possible. Lowers head of bed. Removes the pillow for later use. Locks bed wheels. Raises side rail on far side of bed.

☐ 5. Stands by bed with feet apart, facing client. Places one arm under client's shoulders and the other under client's thighs.

☐ 6. Instructs client to bend knees and push down with his feet on the count of three.

☐ 7. Assists client to move toward the head of the bed on the count of three.

☐ 8. Positions client comfortably, arranges pillow and blankets, and returns bed to lowest position.

☐ 9. Washes hands.

☐ 10. Documents procedure and any observations.

Comments:

If client cannot assist:

☐ 1. Washes hands.

☐ 2. Explains procedure to client, speaking clearly, slowly, and directly. Maintains face-to-face contact whenever possible.

☐ 3. Provides privacy.

□ 4. Adjusts the bed to safe working level, if possible. Lowers head of bed. Removes the pillow for later use. Locks bed wheels. Raises side rail on far side of bed.

□ 5. Stands behind head of bed with feet apart and one foot slightly in front of other.

□ 6. Rolls and grasps top of draw sheet, bends knees, keeping back straight, and rocks weight from front foot to back foot.

□ 7. Positions client comfortably, arranges pillow and blankets, unrolls draw sheet, and returns bed to lowest position.

□ 8. Washes hands.

□ 9. Documents procedure and any observations.

Comments:

When you have help from another person and client cannot assist:

□ 1. Washes hands.

□ 2. Explains procedure to client, speaking clearly, slowly, and directly. Maintains face-to-face contact whenever possible.

□ 3. Provides privacy.

□ 4. Adjusts the bed to safe working level, if possible. Lowers head of bed. Removes the pillow for later use. Locks bed wheels. Raises side rail on far side of bed.

□ 5. Stands on opposite side of bed from helper. Turns slightly toward the head of bed, points foot closest toward head of bed.

□ 6. Rolls and grasps top of draw sheet with palms up.

□ 7. Shifts weight to back foot and on count of three, both workers shift weight to forward feet while sliding draw sheet toward head of bed.

□ 8. Positions client comfortably, arranges pillow and blankets, unrolls draw sheet, and returns bed to lowest position.

□ 9. Washes hands.

□ 10. Documents procedure and any observations.

Comments:

Moving a client to the side of the bed

✓ **Procedure Steps**

□ 1. Washes hands.

□ 2. Explains procedure to client, speaking clearly, slowly, and directly. Maintains face-to-face contact whenever possible.

□ 3. Provides privacy.

□ 4. Adjusts the bed to safe working level, if possible. Locks bed wheels.

□ 5. Stands on same side of bed to where client will be moved.

□ 6. *With a draw sheet*: Rolls draw sheet up and grasps draw sheet with palms up. Puts hand at client's shoulders, and the other at client's hips. Applies one knee against side of bed, leans back and pulls draw sheet and client on the count of three.

Without a draw sheet: Slides hands under head and shoulders and moves toward self. Slides hands under midsection and moves toward self. Slides hands under hips and legs and moves toward self.

□ 7. Returns bed to lowest position.

❑ 8. Washes hands.

❑ 9. Documents procedure and any observations.

Comments:

❑ 9. Returns bed to lowest position if raised.

❑ 10. Washes hands.

❑ 11. Documents procedure and any observations.

Comments:

Turning a client

✓ Procedure Steps

❑ 1. Washes hands.

❑ 2. Explains procedure to client, speaking clearly, slowly, and directly. Maintains face-to-face contact whenever possible.

❑ 3. Provides privacy.

❑ 4. Adjusts the bed to a safe working level, if possible. Locks bed wheels.

❑ 5. Stands at opposite side of the bed to where client will be turned. Raises far side rail and lowers near side rail.

❑ 6. Moves client to side of bed using proper procedure.

Turning client away from you:

❑ 7. Crosses client's arm over chest and crosses leg nearest self over far leg. Stands with feet about 12 inches apart, bends knees and places one hand on client's shoulder and the other on the nearest hip. Pushes client toward other side of bed while shifting weight from back leg to front leg.

Turning client toward you:

❑   Crosses client's arm over chest and crosses leg farthest from self over near leg. Stands with feet about 12 inches apart, bends knees and places one hand on client's far shoulder and the other on the far hip. Rolls client toward self.

❑ 8. Positions client comfortably using pillows or other supports, and checks for good alignment.

Logrolling a client

✓ Procedure Steps

❑ 1. Washes hands.

❑ 2. Explains procedure to client, speaking clearly, slowly, and directly. Maintains face-to-face contact whenever possible.

❑ 3. Provides privacy.

❑ 4. Adjusts the bed to safe working level, if possible. Lowers head of bed. Locks bed wheels. Lowers side rail on side closest to self.

❑ 5. Both workers stand on same side of bed, one at the client's head and shoulders, one near the midsection.

❑ 6. Places client's arm across his chest and places pillow between the knees.

❑ 7. Stands with feet about 12 inches apart, bends knees, and grasps draw sheet on far side.

❑ 8. Rolls client toward self on count of three, turning client as a unit.

❑ 9. Positions client comfortably with pillows or supports, and checks for good alignment. Raises side rail if ordered. Returns bed to lowest position.

❑ 10. Washes hands.

❑ 11. Documents procedure and any observations.

Comments:

Assisting a client to sit up on side of bed: dangling

✓ Procedure Steps

❑ 1. Washes hands.

❑ 2. Explains procedure to client, speaking clearly, slowly, and directly. Maintains face-to-face contact whenever possible.

❑ 3. Provides privacy.

❑ 4. Adjusts the bed to lowest position. Locks bed wheels.

❑ 5. Fanfolds top covers to foot of bed and assists client to turn onto side, facing self.

❑ 6. Has client reach across chest with top arm and place hand on edge of bed near opposite shoulder. Asks client to push down on that hand while swinging legs over the side of bed.

❑ 7. If client needs assistance, stands with legs 12 inches apart, with one foot 6 inches in front of the other. Bends knees.

❑ 8. Places one arm under client's shoulder blades and the other under her thighs.

❑ 9. Turns client into sitting position on count of three.

❑ 10. With client holding onto edge of mattress, puts nonskid shoes on client. Does not leave client alone.

❑ 11. Returns client safely to bed or completes walking or transfer according to care plan.

❑ 12. Washes hands.

❑ 13. Documents procedure and any observations.

Comments:

Transferring a client from a bed to wheelchair

✓ Procedure Steps

❑ 1. Washes hands.

❑ 2. Explains procedure to client, speaking clearly, slowly, and directly. Maintains face-to-face contact whenever possible.

❑ 3. Provides privacy.

❑ 4. Removes footrests and places chair near the head of the bed on client's stronger side. Locks wheelchair wheels.

❑ 5. Raises head of bed and adjusts bed level so that the height of bed is equal to or higher than chair. Locks bed wheels.

❑ 6. Assists client to sitting position with feet flat on floor. Puts non-skid shoes on client and fastens.

❑ 7. *With transfer belt*: Stands in front of client with feet about 12 inches apart. Bends knees. Places transfer belt around client's waist and grasps belt on both sides.

❑ *Without transfer belt*: Stands in front of client with feet about 12 inches apart. Bends knees. Places arms around client's torso under her arms and asks her to place hands on caregiver's shoulders.

❑ 8. Provides instructions to assist with transfer. Braces legs against client's lower legs. Helps client stand on count of three.

❑ 9. Instructs client to take small steps to the chair while turning back toward chair. Assists client to pivot to front of chair if necessary.

❑ 10. Asks client to put hands on chair arm rests and helps client to lower herself into the chair.

❑ 11. Replaces foot rests and places client's feet on them. Positions client comfortably, checking for good alignment and placing robe or blanket over lap.

❏ 12. Washes hands.

❏ 13. Documents procedure and any observations.

Comments:

❏ 12. Washes hands.

❏ 13. Documents procedure and any observations.

Comments:

Helping a client transfer using a slide board

✓ Procedure Steps

❏ 1. Washes hands.

❏ 2. Explains procedure to client, speaking clearly, slowly, and directly. Maintains face-to-face contact whenever possible.

❏ 3. Provides privacy.

❏ 4. Removes footrests and places chair near the head of the bed on client's stronger side. Locks wheelchair wheels.

❏ 5. Raises head of bed and adjusts bed level so that the height of bed is equal to or higher than chair. Locks bed wheels.

❏ 6. Assists client to sitting position with feet flat on floor. Puts non-skid shoes on client and fastens.

❏ 7. Instructs client to lean away from the transfer side.

❏ 8. Places one end of slide board under client's buttocks and thigh and the other end on the surface to which client is transferring.

❏ 9. Instructs client to push up with hands and scoot across the board.

❏ 10. If client needs assistance, braces client's knees, grasps the transfer belt, and instructs client to lean forward. Assists client to scoot across the board, without dragging client.

❏ 11. Removes sliding board after transfer is complete. Positions client comfortably, checking for good alignment.

Transferring a client using a mechanical lift

✓ Procedure Steps

❏ 1. Washes hands.

❏ 2. Explains procedure to client, speaking clearly, slowly, and directly. Maintains face-to-face contact whenever possible.

❏ 3. Provides privacy.

❏ 4. Locks bed wheels. Positions wheelchair next to bed and locks brakes.

❏ 5. Positions sling under client, rolling client to one side of bed and then the other.

❏ 6. Positions mechanical lift next to bed, opening the base to its widest point and pushes base of lift under bed. Positions overhead bar directly over client.

❏ 7. Attaches straps to sling properly.

❏ 8. Raises client in sling two inches above bed, following manufacturer's instructions. Allows client to gain balance.

❏ 9. Rolls mechanical lift to position client over chair or wheelchair. Lifting partner supports and guides client's body.

❏ 10. Slowly lowers client into chair or wheelchair, pushing down gently on client's knees.

❏ 11. Undoes straps from overhead bar to sling, leaving sling in place.

❏ 12. Positions client comfortably, checking for good alignment.

❏ 13. Washes hands.

- ❏ 14. Documents procedure and any observations.

Comments:

Assisting a client to ambulate

✓ Procedure Steps

- ❏ 1. Washes hands.

- ❏ 2. Explains procedure to client, speaking clearly, slowly, and directly. Maintains face-to-face contact whenever possible.

- ❏ 3. Provides privacy.

- ❏ 4. Puts nonskid footwear on client. Adjusts the bed to low position so that feet are flat on the floor. Locks bed wheels.

- ❏ 5. Stands in front of and faces client.

- ❏ 6. Braces client's lower extremities and bends knees.

- ❏ 7. *With transfer belt*: Places belt around client's waist. Bends knees, leans forward, and grasps the belt. Has client lean forward. Rocks weight onto back foot to assist client to standing position on count of three.

- ❏ *Without transfer belt*: Places arms around client's torso under armpits, while assisting client to stand.

- ❏ 8. *With transfer belt*: Walks slightly behind and to one side of client for distance while holding on to transfer belt.

- ❏ *Without transfer belt*: Walks slightly behind and to one side of the client for full distance, supporting client's back with arm. Stands on weaker side.

- ❏ 9. Observes client's strength and provides chair if client becomes tired.

- ❏ 10. Removes transfer belt and returns the client safely to bed or a chair. Positions client comfortably. Returns bed to lowest position.

- ❏ 11. Washes hands.

- ❏ 12. Documents procedure and any observations.

Comments:

Assisting with ambulation for a client who uses a cane, walker or crutches

✓ Procedure Steps

- ❏ 1. Washes hands.

- ❏ 2. Explains procedure to client, speaking clearly, slowly, and directly. Maintains face-to-face contact whenever possible.

- ❏ 3. Provides privacy.

- ❏ 4. Puts nonskid footwear on client. Adjusts the bed to low position so that feet are flat on the floor. Locks bed wheels.

- ❏ 5. Stands in front of and faces client.

- ❏ 6. Braces client's lower extremities and bends knees.

- ❏ 7. Places transfer belt around client's waist and grasps the belt, while assisting client to stand.

- ❏ 8. Helps as needed with ambulation with cane, walker, or crutches, walking slightly behind or on the weak side of client.

- ❏ 9. Watches for obstacles in the client's path.

- ❏ 10. Lets the client set the pace, encouraging rest as necessary.

- ❏ 11. Removes transfer belt. Returns the client safely to bed or a chair and positions client comfortably. Returns bed to lowest position.

- ❏ 12. Washes hands.

- ❏ 13. Documents procedure and any observations.

Comments:

Giving a back rub

✓ Procedure Steps

❏ 1. Washes hands.

❏ 2. Explains procedure to client, speaking clearly, slowly, and directly. Maintains face-to-face contact whenever possible.

❏ 3. Provides privacy.

❏ 4. Adjusts the bed to safe working level, if possible. Lowers head of bed. Locks bed wheels.

❏ 5. Instructs client to lie in prone position or side position. Covers client with blanket and folds back bed covers, exposing client's back to the top of the buttocks.

❏ 6. Warms lotion and hands. Pours lotion onto hands and rubs hands together. Warns client that lotion may still feel cool.

❏ 7. Starting at the upper part of the buttocks, makes long, smooth upward strokes with both hands. Circles hands up along spine, shoulders, and then back down along the outer edges of the back. Repeats for three to five minutes.

❏ 8. Starting at the base of the spine, makes kneading motions using the first two fingers and thumb of each hand. Circles hands up along spine, circling at shoulders and buttocks.

❏ 9. Gently massages bony areas. Massages around any red areas, rather than on them.

❏ 10. Lets client know when back rub is almost completed.

❏ 11. Dries the back and applies powder, if appropriate.

❏ 12. Removes blanket and towel, assists client with getting dressed, and positions client comfortably. Returns bed to lowest position.

❏ 13. Stores lotion and disposes of dirty linens properly.

❏ 14. Washes hands.

❏ 15. Documents procedure and any observations.

Comments:

13

Personal Care Skills

Helping the client transfer to the bathtub

✓ Procedure Steps

❏ 1. Washes hands.

❏ 2. Explains procedure to client, speaking clearly, slowly, and directly. Maintains face-to-face contact whenever possible.

❏ 3. Helps client to the bathroom.

❏ 4. Provides privacy.

❏ 5. Seats client in chair facing tub. If using wheelchair, locks brakes and raises foot rests.

❏ 6. Places client's legs one at a time over sides of tub.

❏ 7. Brings client to sitting position on edge of tub properly.

❏ 8. Lowers client into tub properly, assisting as necessary.

❏ 9. Reverses procedure to help client out of tub.

❏ 10. Washes hands.

❏ 11. Documents procedure and any observations.

Comments:

Helping the ambulatory client take a shower or tub bath

✓ Procedure Steps

❏ 1. Washes hands.

❏ 2. Explains procedure to client, speaking clearly, slowly, and directly. Maintains face-to-face contact whenever possible.

❏ 3. Cleans tub if necessary, places mat, and sets up tub or shower chair. Places non-skid rug next to tub.

❏ 4. Provides privacy.

❏ 5. Puts on gloves if client has broken skin.

❏ 6. Fills tub with warm water (105°F to 110°F on bath thermometer) or adjusts shower water temperature. Has client test water temperature and adjusts as necessary.

❏ 7. Assists client to undress as necessary and helps client to tub or shower.

❏ 8. If client is able to bathe alone, places supplies and signal near client. Checks on client every five minutes. If client is weak, stays in bathroom.

❏ 9. If showering, stays with client and assists.

❏ 10. Assists client as necessary, washing from clean to dirty areas. Assists with rinsing thoroughly.

❏ 11. Assists with shampooing.

❏ 12. Helps client out and assists client with drying if necessary.

❏ 13. Helps client to bed.

❏ 14. Cleans tub. Places soiled laundry in laundry hamper.

❏ 15. Washes hands.

❏ 16. Puts supplies away.

❏ 17. Documents procedure and any observations.

Comments:

Giving a complete bed bath

✓ Procedure Steps

❏ 1. Washes hands.

❏ 2. Explains procedure to client, speaking clearly, slowly, and directly. Maintains face-to-face contact whenever possible.

❏ 3. Provides privacy.

❏ 4. Adjusts the bed to a safe working level, if possible. Locks bed wheels.

❏ 5. Asks client to remove glasses and jewelry. Offers bedpan.

❏ 6. Places blanket over client and checks sheets.

❏ 7. Fills basin and checks temperature (105°F to 110°F). Has client test water temperature and adjusts if necessary.

❏ 8. Puts on gloves if client has open lesions or wounds.

❏ 9. Asks and assists client to participate in washing.

❏ 10. Uncovers only one part of the body at a time. Places a towel under the body part being washed.

❏ 11. Washes, rinses, and dries one part of the body at a time. Starts at the head, working down, and completing front first.

Eyes and Face:

❏ Washes face with wet washcloth (no soap) beginning with the eyes, using a different area of the washcloth for each eye, washing inner aspect to outer aspect. Washes the face from the middle outward using firm but gentle strokes. Washes neck and ears and behind the ears. Rinses and pats dry.

Arms and Hands:

❏ Washes arm and underarm. Uses long strokes from the shoulder down to the elbow. Rinses and pats dry. Washes the elbow. Washes, rinses, and dries from the elbow down to the wrist.

❏ Cleans under nails. Rinses and pats dry. Gives nail care. Washes hand in a basin. Provides nail care if it has been assigned. Repeats for other arm and hand. Applies lotion if ordered.

Chest:

❏ Lifts the towel only enough to wash the chest, rinse it, and pat dry. For a female client: washes, rinses, and dries breasts and under breasts.

Abdomen:

❏ Washes abdomen, rinses and pats dry.

Legs and Feet:

❏ Washes the thigh. Uses long downward strokes. Rinses and pats dry. Does the same from the knee to the ankle.

❏ Washes the foot and between the toes in a basin. Rinses foot and pats dry, making sure area between toes is dry. Provides nail care if it has been assigned. Applies lotion if ordered but not between the toes.

Back:

❏ Helps client move to the center of the bed, then turns onto his side so back is facing self. Washes back, neck, and buttocks with long, downward strokes. Rinses and pats dry. Applies lotion if ordered.

❏ 12. Puts on gloves before washing perineal area.

❏ 13. Changes bath water. Washes, rinses, and dries perineal area, working from front to back.

For a female client:

❏ Washes the perineum with soap and water from front to back, using single strokes. Uses a clean area of washcloth or clean washcloth for each stroke. Wipes the center of the perineum, then each side. Spreads the labia majora. Wipes from front to back on each side. Rinses the area in the same way. Dries entire

perineal area moving from front to back, using a blotting motion with towel. Asks client to turn on her side. Washes, rinses, and dries buttocks and anal area. Cleanses anal area without contaminating the perineal area.

For a male client:

❏ If client is uncircumcised, retracts the foreskin first. Gently pushes skin towards the base of penis. Holds the penis by the shaft and washes in a circular motion from the tip down to the base. Uses a clean area of washcloth or clean washcloth for each stroke. Rinses the penis. If client is uncircumcised, gently returns foreskin to normal position. Then washes the scrotum and groin. Rinses and pats dry. Asks client to turn on his side. Washes, rinses, and dries buttocks and anal area. Cleanses anal area without contaminating the perineal area.

❏ 14. Covers client. Disposes of water and gloves properly. Places soiled washcloths and towels in proper container.

❏ 15. Gives back rub if time permits.

❏ 16. Assist client with grooming as necessary. Returns bed to lowest position.

❏ 17. Washes and stores everything. Changes bed sheets and blankets.

❏ 18. Washes hands.

❏ 19. Documents procedure and any observations.

Comments:

Shampooing hair

✓ Procedure Steps

❏ 1. Washes hands.

❏ 2. Explains procedure to client, speaking clearly, slowly, and directly. Maintains face-to-face contact whenever possible.

❑ 3. Provides privacy.

❑ 4. Positions client in sink, tub, shower, or in bed, and wets hair.

❑ 5. Applies shampoo, and massages scalp.

❑ 6. Rinses hair. Repeats.

❑ 7. Wraps client's hair.

❑ 8. Removes towel and combs/brushes hair.

❑ 9. Dries and styles hair.

❑ 10. Washes and stores equipment. Removes gloves.

❑ 11. Washes hands.

❑ 12. Documents procedure and any observations.

Comments:

Providing fingernail care

✓ Procedure Steps

❑ 1. Washes hands.

❑ 2. Explains procedure to client, speaking clearly, slowly, and directly. Maintains face-to-face contact whenever possible.

❑ 3. Provides privacy.

❑ 4. Adjusts the bed to a safe working level, if possible. Locks bed wheels.

❑ 5. Removes nail polish if necessary.

❑ 6. Fills basin with warm water (105°F). Has client test water temperature and adjusts if necessary.

❑ 7. Soaks the client's nails for two to four minutes.

❑ 8. Removes hands from water. Washes hands with soapy washcloth. Rinses. Dries client's hands with a towel, including between fingers.

❑ 9. Puts on gloves.

❑ 10. Cleans under nails with orangewood stick. Wipes orangewood stick on towel after each nail. Washes the hands again and dries.

❑ 11. Shapes fingernails with an emery board or nail file. Finishes with nails free of rough edges. Applies lotion.

❑ 12. Discards water and cleans basin. Disposes of towels in proper place and stores supplies. Discards gloves. Returns bed to lowest position.

❑ 13. Washes hands.

❑ 14. Documents procedure and any observations.

Comments:

Providing foot care

✓ Procedure Steps

❑ 1. Washes hands.

❑ 2. Explains procedure to client, speaking clearly, slowly, and directly. Maintains face-to-face contact whenever possible.

❑ 3. Provides privacy.

❑ 4. Fills basin with warm water (105°F). Has client test water temperature and adjusts if necessary.

❑ 5. Soaks client's feet for five to ten minutes, adding warm water as necessary.

❑ 6. Puts on gloves.

❑ 7. Removes one foot from water. Washes entire foot, including between the toes and around nail beds with soapy washcloth.

❑ 8. Rinses and dries entire foot, including between the toes, with a soapy washcloth. Applies lotion.

❑ 9. Repeats steps for other foot.

❏ 10. Observes condition of feet.

❏ 11. Assists client to replace socks.

❏ 12. Discards water and cleans basin. Disposes of towels properly. Discards gloves.

❏ 13. Washes hands.

❏ 14. Documents procedure and any observations.

Comments:

Shaving a client

✓ Procedure Steps

❏ 1. Washes hands.

❏ 2. Explains procedure to client, speaking clearly, slowly, and directly. Maintains face-to-face contact whenever possible.

❏ 3. Provides privacy.

❏ 4. Places equipment within reach. Adjust beds to a safe working level, if possible. Locks bed wheels. Places towel across client's chest.

❏ 5. Puts on gloves.

❏ 6. *If using a safety or disposable razor*, softens beard, lathers face, and shaves in direction of hair growth. Rinses blade often. Rinses and dries face. Offers mirror.

❏ *If using an electric razor*, cleans it. Turns on, pulls skin taut, and shaves with smooth, even movements. Shaves beard with back and forth motion in direction of beard growth with foil shaver. Shaves beard in circular motion with three-head shaver. Shaves the chin and under the chin. Offers mirror.

❏ 7. Applies aftershave if client desires.

❏ 8. Puts towel and linens in hamper. Removes and discards gloves. Returns bed to lowest position. Cleans and stores equipment.

❏ 9. Washes hands.

❏ 10. Documents procedure and any observations.

Comments:

Combing or brushing hair

✓ Procedure Steps

❏ 1. Washes hands.

❏ 2. Explains procedure to client, speaking clearly, slowly, and directly. Maintains face-to-face contact whenever possible.

❏ 3. Provides privacy.

❏ 4. If confined to bed, raises head and places towel under it. Adjusts the bed to a safe working level, if possible. Locks bed wheels. If ambulatory, provides comfortable chair. Places towel under head or around shoulders.

❏ 5. Removes hairpins, hair ties, and clips.

❏ 6. If hair is tangled, detangles gently.

❏ 7. Brushes hair properly.

❏ 8. Styles hair in the way the client prefers. Offers a mirror to client.

❏ 9. Removes towel, and places linen in hamper. Cleans and stores supplies. Returns bed to lowest position.

❏ 10. Washes hands.

❏ 11. Documents procedure and any observations.

Comments:

Providing oral care

✓ **Procedure Steps**

☐ 1. Washes hands.

☐ 2. Explains procedure to client, speaking clearly, slowly, and directly. Maintains face-to-face contact whenever possible.

☐ 3. Provides privacy.

☐ 4. If client is in bed, helps him into upright sitting position. Adjusts the bed to a safe working level, if possible. Locks bed wheels.

☐ 5. Puts on gloves. Places towel under head and across chest.

☐ 6. Removes dental bridgework.

☐ 7. Wets brush and puts a small amount of toothpaste on brush.

☐ 8. Gently brushes teeth, including tongue and all surfaces of teeth.

☐ 9. Rinses mouth and allows client to spit.

☐ 10. Wipes client's mouth and removes towel.

☐ 11. Replaces dental bridgework. Applies moisturizer to lips.

☐ 12. Disposes of water, washes and stores equipment. Removes gloves. Returns bed to lowest position.

☐ 13. Washes hands.

☐ 14. Documents procedure and any observations.

Comments:

Providing oral care for the unconscious client

✓ **Procedure Steps**

☐ 1. Washes hands.

☐ 2. Explains procedure to client, speaking clearly, slowly, and directly. Maintains face-to-face contact whenever possible.

☐ 3. Provides privacy.

☐ 4. Adjusts the bed to a safe working level, if possible. Locks bed wheels.

☐ 5. Puts on gloves.

☐ 6. Turns client's head and places a towel under cheek and chin. Places basin next to cheek and chin.

☐ 7. Separates upper and lower teeth with padded tongue blade. Swabs teeth, gums, tongue, and inside surfaces of mouth. Repeats until clean.

☐ 8. Rinses with clean swab.

☐ 9. Removes towel and basin. Applies moisturizer to lips.

☐ 10. Washes and stores supplies. Removes and discards gloves. Returns bed to lowest position.

☐ 11. Washes hands.

☐ 12. Documents procedure and any observations.

Comments:

Flossing teeth

✓ **Procedure Steps**

☐ 1. Washes hands.

☐ 2. Explains procedure to client, speaking clearly, slowly, and directly. Maintains face-to-face contact whenever possible.

☐ 3. Provides privacy.

☐ 4. Helps client get into upright sitting position. Adjusts the bed to safe working level, if possible. Locks bed wheels.

☐ 5. Puts on gloves.

☐ 6. Wraps floss around fingers.

☐ 7. Flosses teeth, starting with back and moving to gum line.

❏ 8. Uses clean area of floss after every two teeth.

❏ 9. Offers water periodically and offers a towel when done.

❏ 10. Washes and stores supplies. Removes gloves. Returns bed to lowest position.

❏ 11. Washes hands.

❏ 12. Documents procedure and any observations.

Comments:

Cleaning and storing dentures

✓ **Procedure Steps**

❏ 1. Washes hands.

❏ 2. Explains procedure to client, speaking clearly, slowly, and directly. Maintains face-to-face contact whenever possible.

❏ 3. Provides privacy.

❏ 4. Lines sink or basin with towel and fills with water.

❏ 5. Puts on gloves.

❏ 6. Removes lower denture properly if client is unable.

❏ 7. Removes upper denture properly.

❏ 8. Applies denture cleanser to toothbrush and brushes all surfaces. Rinses all surfaces under cool running water.

❏ 9. Rinses denture cup and places dentures in it.

❏ 10. If client prefers, soaks dentures in solution.

❏ 11. Stores dentures in water or solution in labeled denture cup.

❏ 12. Washes and stores supplies. Removes and discards gloves.

❏ 13. Washes hands.

❏ 14. Documents procedure and any observations.

Comments:

Reinserting dentures

✓ **Procedure Steps**

❏ 1. Washes hands.

❏ 2. Explains procedure to client, speaking clearly, slowly, and directly. Maintains face-to-face contact whenever possible.

❏ 3. Provides privacy.

❏ 4. Positions client in upright position.

❏ 5. Puts on gloves.

❏ 6. Applies denture cream.

❏ 7. Inserts upper denture at an angle, pressing it firmly onto upper gum line.

❏ 8. Inserts lower denture, pressing it firmly onto the lower gum line.

❏ 9. Offers client face towel.

❏ 10. Rinses and stores denture cup. Removes and discards gloves.

❏ 11. Washes hands.

❏ 12. Documents procedure and any observations.

Comments:

Assisting a client with use of a bedpan

✓ **Procedure Steps**

❏ 1. Washes hands.

❏ 2. Explains procedure to client, speaking clearly, slowly, and directly. Maintains face-to-face contact whenever possible.

❏ 3. Provides privacy.

❑ 4. Adjusts the bed to a safe working level, if possible. Locks bed wheels. Lowers head of bed.

❑ 5. Puts on gloves.

❑ 6. Warms outside of bedpan with warm water. Dusts it with talcum powder.

❑ 7. Covers client with bath blanket. Places a protective sheet under client properly.

❑ 8. Asks client to remove undergarments or assists client to do so.

❑ 9. Slides bedpan under hips, helping client if necessary. Raise head of bed after placing bedpan.

❑ 10. Checks bedpan position, ensuring blanket is covering client. Provides client with supplies and leaves room until client calls.

❑ 11. When called, returns and lowers head of bed. Removes and covers bedpan. If client is unable, cleans the perineum properly.

❑ 12. Discards soiled supplies properly. Dries perineal area. Removes and discards gloves.

❑ 13. Puts on new gloves properly.

❑ 14. Offers washcloth and soap to client to wash hands. Covers client and helps put on undergarments.

❑ 15. Empties bedpan into toilet.

❑ 16. Rinses bedpan with cold water and empties. Cleans bedpan with hot, soapy water.

❑ 17. Removes and discards gloves.

❑ 18. Washes hands. Returns bed to lowest position.

❑ 19. Documents procedure and any observations.

Comments:

Assisting a male client with a urinal
✓ **Procedure Steps**

❑ 1. Washes hands.

❑ 2. Explains procedure to client, speaking clearly, slowly, and directly. Maintains face-to-face contact whenever possible.

❑ 3. Provides privacy.

❑ 4. Adjusts the bed to a safe working level, if possible. Locks bed wheels.

❑ 5. Puts on gloves.

❑ 6. Places protective pad under buttocks and hips.

❑ 7. Hands urinal to client or places it if client is unable. Replaces covers.

❑ 8. Leaves room, giving client a bell.

❑ 9. Removes urinal when client is finished.

❑ 10. Discards urine and rinses urinal and stores.

❑ 11. Removes and discards gloves. Washes hands.

❑ 12. Gives client washcloth, soap, and water to wash his hands.

❑ 13. After discarding supplies, washes hands again. Returns bed to lowest position.

❑ 14. Documents procedure and any observations.

Comments:

Assisting a client in using a portable commode or toilet
✓ **Procedure Steps**

❑ 1. Washes hands.

❑ 2. Explains procedure to client, speaking clearly, slowly, and directly. Maintains face-to-face contact whenever possible.

❑ 3. Provides privacy.

❏ 4. Adjusts the bed to a safe working level, if possible. Locks bed wheels.

❏ 5. Puts on gloves.

❏ 6. Helps client to bathroom or commode.

❏ 7. Leaves room or area, giving client a bell to call.

❏ 8. Returns when client is done. Cleans perineal area if assistance is needed.

❏ 9. Helps client up and ensures client's hands are washed.

❏ 10. Removes waste container and empties into toilet.

❏ 11. Cleans container, rinsing first with cold water, then hot.

❏ 12. Removes gloves and discards them. Returns bed to lowest position.

❏ 13. Washes hands.

❏ 14. Documents procedure and any observations.

Comments:

14

Core Healthcare Skills

Taking and recording an oral temperature

✓ Procedure Steps

❏ 1. Washes hands.

❏ 2. Explains procedure to client, speaking clearly, slowly, and directly. Maintains face-to-face contact whenever possible.

❏ 3. Provides privacy.

Mercury-free thermometer:

❏ 4. Holds thermometer by stem. Shakes thermometer down to below the lowest number.

Digital thermometer:

❏ Puts on disposable sheath. Turns on thermometer and waits until "ready" sign appears.

Electronic thermometer:

❏ Removes probe from base unit and puts on probe cover.

Mercury-free thermometer:

❏ 5. Puts on disposable sheath, if available. Inserts bulb end of thermometer into client's mouth, under tongue and to one side.

Digital thermometer:

❏ Inserts end of digital thermometer into client's mouth, under tongue and to one side.

Electronic thermometer:

❏ Inserts end of electronic thermometer into client's mouth, under tongue and to one side.

Mercury-free thermometer:

❏ 6. Instructs client on how to hold thermometer in mouth. Leaves thermometer in place for at least three minutes.

Digital thermometer:

❏ Leaves in place until thermometer blinks or beeps.

Electronic thermometer:

❏ Leaves in place until tone or light signals temperature has been read.

Mercury-free thermometer:

❏ 7. Removes thermometer. Wipes with tissue from stem to bulb or removes sheath. Disposes of tissue or sheath. Reads temperature and remembers reading.

Digital thermometer:

❏ Removes thermometer. Reads temperature on display screen and remembers reading.

Electronic thermometer:

❑ Reads temperature on display screen and remembers reading.

Mercury-free thermometer:

❑ 8. Rinses and dries thermometer and stores properly.

Digital thermometer:

❑ Removes and disposes of sheath with a tissue. Stores thermometer.

Electronic thermometer:

❑ Presses the eject button to discard the cover. Returns probe to holder.

❑ 9. Removes and discards gloves.

❑ 10. Washes hands.

❑ 11. Documents temperature, date, time and method used.

Comments:

Taking and recording a rectal temperature

✓ Procedure Steps

❑ 1. Washes hands.

❑ 2. Explains procedure to client, speaking clearly, slowly, and directly. Maintains face-to-face contact whenever possible.

❑ 3. Provides privacy.

❑ 4. Assists client to left-lying position.

❑ 5. Folds back linens to only expose rectal area.

❑ 6. Puts on gloves.

Mercury-free thermometer:

❑ 7. Holds thermometer by stem. Shakes thermometer down to below the lowest number.

Digital thermometer:

❑ Puts on disposable sheath. Turns on thermometer and waits until "ready" sign appears.

❑ 8. Applies a small amount of lubricant to tip or bulb or probe cover.

❑ 9. Separates buttocks. Gently inserts thermometer into rectum one inch. Replaces sheet over buttocks. Holds onto thermometer at all times while taking temperature.

Mercury-free thermometer:

❑ 10. Holds thermometer in place for at least three minutes.

Digital thermometer:

❑ Holds thermometer in place until thermometer blinks or beeps.

❑ 11. Removes thermometer and wipes thermometer with tissue from stem to bulb or removes sheath. Disposes of tissue or sheath.

❑ 12. Reads temperature and remembers reading.

Mercury-free thermometer:

❑ 13. Rinses and dries thermometer and stores properly.

Digital thermometer:

❑ Stores thermometer.

❑ 14. Removes and discards gloves.

❑ 15. Washes hands.

❑ 16. Documents temperature, date, time and method used.

Comments:

Taking and recording a tympanic temperature

✓ Procedure Steps

❑ 1. Washes hands.

❑ 2. Explains procedure to client, speaking clearly, slowly, and directly. Maintains face-to-face contact whenever possible.

❑ 3. Provides privacy.

❑ 4. Puts on gloves.

❑ 5. Places disposable sheath over earpiece of thermometer.

❑ 6. Positions client's head properly and pulls up and back on the outside edge of the ear. Inserts covered probe and presses the button.

❑ 7. Holds thermometer in place for one second or until it beeps.

❑ 8. Reads temperature and remembers reading.

❑ 9. Discards sheath and stores thermometer properly.

❑ 10. Removes and discards gloves.

❑ 11. Washes hands.

❑ 12. Documents temperature, date, time and method used.

Comments:

Taking and recording an axillary temperature

✓ Procedure Steps

❑ 1. Washes hands.

❑ 2. Explains procedure to client, speaking clearly, slowly, and directly. Maintains face-to-face contact whenever possible.

❑ 3. Provides privacy.

❑ 4. Puts on gloves.

❑ 5. Adjusts client's clothing as necessary and makes sure axilla is dry.

Mercury-free thermometer:

❑ 6. Holds thermometer by stem. Shakes thermometer down to below the lowest number.

Digital thermometer:

❑ Puts on disposable sheath. Turns on thermometer and waits until "ready" sign appears.

Electronic thermometer:

❑ Removes probe from base unit and puts on probe cover.

❑ 7. Positions thermometer in center of armpit and folds client's arm over chest.

Mercury-free thermometer:

❑ 8. Holds thermometer in place for eight to ten minutes.

Digital thermometer:

❑ Leaves in place until thermometer blinks or beeps.

Electronic thermometer:

❑ Leaves in place until tone or light signals temperature has been read.

Mercury-free thermometer:

❑ 9. Removes thermometer. Wipes with tissue from stem to bulb or removes sheath. Disposes of tissue or sheath. Reads temperature and remembers reading.

Digital thermometer:

❑ Removes thermometer. Reads temperature on display screen and remembers reading.

Electronic thermometer:

❑ Reads temperature on display screen and remembers reading.

Mercury-free thermometer:

❑ 10. Rinses and dries thermometer and stores properly.

Digital thermometer:

- ☐ Removes and disposes of sheath with a tissue. Stores thermometer.

Electronic thermometer:

- ☐ Presses the eject button to discard the cover. Returns probe to holder.
- ☐ 11. Removes and discards gloves.
- ☐ 12. Washes hands.
- ☐ 13. Documents temperature, date, time and method used.

Comments:

Taking and recording apical pulse

✓ **Procedure Steps**

- ☐ 1. Washes hands.
- ☐ 2. Explains procedure to client, speaking clearly, slowly, and directly. Maintains face-to-face contact whenever possible.
- ☐ 3. Provides privacy.
- ☐ 4. Fits earpieces of stethoscope snugly in ears and places metal diaphragm on left side of chest, just below the nipple.
- ☐ 5. Counts heartbeats for one minute.
- ☐ 6. Counts client's respirations with stethoscope still in place.
- ☐ 7. Documents pulse rate, date, time, and method used. Notes any irregularities in rhythm.
- ☐ 8. Stores stethoscope.
- ☐ 9. Washes hands.

Comments:

Taking and recording radial pulse and counting and recording respirations

✓ **Procedure Steps**

- ☐ 1. Washes hands.
- ☐ 2. Explains procedure to client, speaking clearly, slowly, and directly. Maintains face-to-face contact whenever possible.
- ☐ 3. Provides privacy.
- ☐ 4. Places fingertips on the thumb side of client's wrist to locate pulse.
- ☐ 5. Counts beats for one full minute.
- ☐ 6. Keeping fingertips on client's wrist, counts respirations for one full minute.
- ☐ 7. Documents pulse rate, date, time, and method used. Documents respiratory rate and the pattern or character of breathing.
- ☐ 8. Washes hands.

Comments:

Taking and recording blood pressure (two-step method)

✓ **Procedure Steps**

- ☐ 1. Washes hands.
- ☐ 2. Explains procedure to client, speaking clearly, slowly, and directly. Maintains face-to-face contact whenever possible.
- ☐ 3. Provides privacy.
- ☐ 4. Asks client to roll up sleeve. Positions client's arm with palm up. The arm should be level with the heart.
- ☐ 5. With the valve open, squeezes the cuff to make sure it is completely deflated.
- ☐ 6. Places blood pressure cuff snugly on client's upper arm, with the center of the cuff placed over the brachial artery.

❏ 7. Locates the radial (wrist) pulse with fingertips.

❏ 8. Closes the valve (clockwise) until it stops. Inflates cuff, watching gauge.

❏ 9. Stops inflating cuff when pulse is no longer felt. Notes the reading.

❏ 10. Opens the valve to deflate cuff completely.

❏ 11. Writes down the estimated systolic reading.

❏ 12. Wipes diaphragm and earpieces of stethoscope with alcohol wipes.

❏ 13. Locates brachial pulse with fingertips.

❏ 14. Places earpieces of stethoscope in ears and places diaphragm of stethoscope over brachial artery.

❏ 15. Closes the valve (clockwise) until it stops. Does not tighten it.

❏ 16. Inflates cuff to 30 mmHg above the estimated systolic pressure.

❏ 17. Opens the valve slightly with thumb and index finger. Deflates cuff slowly.

❏ 18. Watches gauge and listens for sound of pulse.

❏ 19. Remembers the reading at which the first clear pulse sound is heard. This is the systolic pressure.

❏ 20. Continues listening for a change or muffling of pulse sound. The point of a change or the point the sound disappears is the diastolic pressure. Remembers this reading.

❏ 21. Opens the valve to deflate cuff completely. Removes cuff.

❏ 22. Documents both systolic and diastolic pressures. Notes which arm was used.

❏ 23. Cleans stethoscope. Stores equipment.

❏ 24. Washes hands.

Comments:

Measuring and recording weight of an ambulatory client

✓ Procedure Steps

❏ 1. Washes hands.

❏ 2. Explains procedure to client, speaking clearly, slowly, and directly. Maintains face-to-face contact whenever possible.

❏ 3. Provides privacy.

❏ 4. Sets scale on hard floor surface and makes sure it reads zero.

❏ 5. Assists client to the scale as necessary.

❏ 6. Instructs client to step on scale, assisting as necessary. Makes sure client is not holding, touching, or leaning against anything.

❏ 7. Determines client's weight. If using a bathroom scale, reads weight when dial has stopped moving. If using a standing scale, balances the bar and adds numbers together.

❏ 8. Assists client to step off the scale and back to a comfortable position.

❏ 9. Documents the weight.

❏ 10. Stores the scale.

❏ 11. Washes hands.

Comments:

Measuring and recording height of a client

✓ Procedure Steps

❏ 1. Washes hands.

☐ 2. Explains procedure to client, speaking clearly, slowly, and directly. Maintains face-to-face contact whenever possible.

☐ 3. Provides privacy.

☐ 4. Positions client in bed, flat on the back, with arms and legs at sides. Makes sure bed sheet is smooth underneath client.

☐ 5. Makes a small pencil mark at the top of client's head and at client's heel.

☐ 6. Measures distance between the two marks with a tape measure.

☐ 7. Documents client's height.

☐ 8. Stores equipment.

☐ 9. Washes hands.

For clients who can get out of bed:

☐ 1. Washes hands.

☐ 2. Explains procedure to client, speaking clearly, slowly, and directly. Maintains face-to-face contact whenever possible.

☐ 3. Provides privacy.

☐ 4. Instructs client to remove shoes and stand with his back against a wall and arms at his sides.

☐ 5. Makes a small pencil mark on the wall even with the top of the client's head.

☐ 6. Instructs client to step away. Measures the distance between the pencil mark and the floor.

☐ 7. Documents height.

☐ 8. Stores equipment.

☐ 9. Washes hands.

If using a standing scale:

☐ 1. Washes hands.

☐ 2. Explains procedure to client, speaking clearly, slowly, and directly. Maintains face-to-face contact whenever possible.

☐ 3. Provides privacy.

☐ 4. Helps client to step onto scale, facing away from the scale.

☐ 5. With client standing straight, pulls up measuring rod and lowers it until it rests flat on client's head.

☐ 6. Determines client's height. Assists client to step off the scale and back to a comfortable position.

☐ 7. Documents the height.

☐ 8. Washes hands.

Comments:

Collecting a sputum specimen

✓ **Procedure Steps**

☐ 1. Washes hands.

☐ 2. Explains procedure to client, speaking clearly, slowly, and directly. Maintains face-to-face contact whenever possible.

☐ 3. Provides privacy.

☐ 4. Puts on mask and gloves.

☐ 5. Gives client tissues to cover the mouth. Instructs client to cough deeply and spit the sputum into the specimen container.

☐ 6. Covers container tightly, and wipes any sputum off the outside of the container. Puts container in plastic bag, and seals it.

☐ 7. Removes and discards gloves and mask.

☐ 8. Washes hands.

☐ 9. Documents procedure and any observations.

Comments:

Collecting a stool specimen

✓ Procedure Steps

❏ 1. Washes hands.

❏ 2. Explains procedure to client, speaking clearly, slowly, and directly. Maintains face-to-face contact whenever possible.

❏ 3. Provides privacy.

❏ 4. Puts on gloves.

❏ 5. Asks client not to urinate at the same time as moving bowels and not to put toilet paper in with the sample. Provides plastic bag to discard toilet paper separately.

❏ 6. Fits hat to toilet or provides client with bedpan. Leaves the room and asks the client to call when he is finished.

❏ 7. Assists as necessary with perineal care. Helps client wash hands, and makes client comfortable. Removes gloves.

❏ 8. Washes hands again.

❏ 9. Puts on clean gloves.

❏ 10. Uses tongue blades to take about two tablespoons of stool and puts it in container without touching the inside. Covers container tightly.

❏ 11. Disposes of tongue blades properly. Empties bedpan or container into toilet. Cleans and stores equipment properly.

❏ 12. Stores the specimen properly.

❏ 13. Removes and discards gloves.

❏ 14. Washes hands.

❏ 15. Documents procedure and any observations.

Comments:

Collecting a routine urine specimen

✓ Procedure Steps

❏ 1. Washes hands.

❏ 2. Explains procedure to client, speaking clearly, slowly, and directly. Maintains face-to-face contact whenever possible.

❏ 3. Provides privacy.

❏ 4. Puts on gloves.

❏ 5. Assists client to bathroom or commode, or offers bedpan or urinal.

❏ 6. Has client void. Asks client not to put toilet paper in with the sample. Provide a plastic bag to discard toilet paper separately.

❏ 7. Assists as necessary with perineal care. Helps client wash his or her hands. Makes client comfortable.

❏ 8. Takes bedpan, urinal, or commode pail to the bathroom.

❏ 9. Pours urine into specimen container, making it at least half full.

❏ 10. Covers container with lid. Wipes off the outside with a paper towel.

❏ 11. Places the container in a plastic bag.

❏ 12. Discards extra urine. Rinses and cleans equipment, and stores it.

❏ 13. Removes and discards gloves.

❏ 14. Washes hands.

❏ 15. Documents procedure and any observations.

Comments:

Collecting a clean catch (mid-stream) urine specimen

✓ Procedure Steps

❏ 1. Washes hands.

❑ 2. Explains procedure to client, speaking clearly, slowly, and directly. Maintains face-to-face contact whenever possible.

❑ 3. Provides privacy.

❑ 4. Puts on gloves.

❑ 5. Opens specimen kit.

❑ 6. Cleans the area around the urethra.

❑ 7. Asks client to urinate into the bedpan, urinal, or toilet, and to stop before urination is complete.

❑ 8. Places container under the urine stream and instructs client to start urinating again until container is at least half full.

❑ 9. Covers urine container and wipes off outside with paper towel. Places in a plastic bag.

❑ 10. Discards extra urine. Rinses, cleans, and stores equipment.

❑ 11. Assist as necessary with perineal care. Removes gloves and washes hands. Assists client to wash hands.

❑ 12. Washes hands again.

❑ 13. Documents procedure and any observations.

Comments:

Collecting a 24-hour urine specimen

✓ **Procedure Steps**

❑ 1. Washes hands.

❑ 2. Explains procedure to client, speaking clearly, slowly, and directly. Maintains face-to-face contact whenever possible.

❑ 3. Provides privacy.

❑ 4. Instructs client to completely empty the bladder. Discards urine and notes the exact time.

❑ 5. Labels container.

❑ 6. Puts on gloves each time client voids.

❑ 7. Pours urine into container using the funnel as needed.

❑ 8. Assists client with perineal care and to wash hands after each voiding.

❑ 9. Instructs family to save all urine and store properly after each voiding.

❑ 10. Cleans equipment after each voiding.

❑ 11. Removes gloves.

❑ 12. Washes hands.

❑ 13. Documents procedure and any observations.

Comments:

Measuring and recording intake and output

✓ **Procedure Steps**

❑ 1. Washes hands.

❑ 2. Explains procedure to client, speaking clearly, slowly, and directly. Maintains face-to-face contact whenever possible.

❑ 3. Provides privacy.

❑ 4. Measures amount of fluid client is served and notes on paper, not visit notes.

❑ 5. Measures leftover fluids and notes on paper, not visit notes.

❑ 6. Subtracts amount left over from amount served. Converts to milliliters.

❑ 7. Documents amount of fluids consumed (in mL), time, and what fluid was taken in visit notes.

For measuring the client's output:

❑ 1. Washes hands.

❏ 2. Explains procedure to client, speaking clearly, slowly, and directly. Maintains face-to-face contact whenever possible.

❏ 3. Provides privacy.

❏ 4. Puts on gloves.

❏ 5. Pours urine into measuring container. Measures amount of urine and notes amount on paper.

❏ 6. Discards urine. Washes and stores equipment properly.

❏ 7. Removes and discards gloves.

❏ 8. Washes hands.

❏ 9. Documents the time and amount (in mL) of urine.

Comments:

Observing, reporting, and documenting emesis

✓ **Procedure Steps**

❏ 1. Puts on gloves.

❏ 2. Provides a basin and removes it when vomiting has stopped.

❏ 3. Removes soiled linens or clothes and replaces with fresh ones.

❏ 4. Measures and notes amount of vomitus, if monitoring client's I&O.

❏ 5. Discards vomit in toilet and washes and stores basin properly.

❏ 6. Removes and discards gloves.

❏ 7. Washes hands.

❏ 8. Puts on fresh gloves.

❏ 9. Provides comfort to client.

❏ 10. Launders soiled linens and clothes in hot water.

❏ 11. Removes and discards gloves.

❏ 12. Washes hands again.

❏ 13. Documents time, amount, color, and consistency of vomitus. Observes for blood.

❏ 14. Reports to supervisor immediately.

Comments:

Providing catheter care

✓ **Procedure Steps**

❏ 1. Washes hands.

❏ 2. Explains procedure to client, speaking clearly, slowly, and directly. Maintains face-to-face contact whenever possible.

❏ 3. Provides privacy.

❏ 4. Adjusts the bed to safe working level, if possible. Locks bed wheels. Lowers head of bed and positions client lying flat on back.

❏ 5. Removes or folds back top bedding, keeping client covered with bath blanket.

❏ 6. Makes sure water temperature is 105° to 109° F.

❏ 7. Puts on gloves.

❏ 8. Places clean protective pad under buttocks.

❏ 9. Exposes only the area necessary to clean the catheter.

❏ 10. Places towel or pad under catheter tubing before washing.

❏ 11. Applies soap to washcloth and cleans area around meatus, using a clean area of the cloth for each stroke.

❏ 12. Holding catheter near meatus, cleans at least four inches of catheter. Moves in only one direction, away from meatus. Uses a clean area of the cloth for each stroke.

13. Rinses area around meatus and rinses at least four inches of catheter nearest meatus, moving away from meatus.

14. Removes towel or pad and bath blanket, and replaces top covers. Empties water into toilet. Disposes of linen in proper containers.

15. Removes and discards gloves. Returns bed to lowest position.

16. Washes hands.

17. Helps client dress. Arranges covers. Checks that catheter tubing is free from kinks and twists and that it is securely taped to the leg.

18. Washes hands again.

19. Documents procedure and any observations.

Comments:

Emptying the catheter drainage bag

✓ **Procedure Steps**

1. Washes hands.

2. Explains procedure to client, speaking clearly, slowly, and directly. Maintains face-to-face contact whenever possible.

3. Puts on gloves.

4. Places measuring container on paper towel on floor.

5. Opens drain or spout on bag so urine flows into measuring container.

6. Closes spout and cleans it. Replaces drain in its holder on the bag.

7. Notes amount and appearance of urine and empties it into toilet.

8. Cleans and stores measuring container properly.

9. Removes and discards gloves.

10. Washes hands.

11. Documents procedure and any observations.

Comments:

Applying a condom catheter

✓ **Procedure Steps**

1. Washes hands.

2. Explains procedure to client, speaking clearly, slowly, and directly. Maintains face-to-face contact whenever possible.

3. Provides privacy.

4. Adjusts the bed to a safe working level, if possible. Locks bed wheels. Lowers head of bed and positions client lying flat on back.

5. Removes or folds back bedding, keeping client covered with bath blanket.

6. Puts on gloves.

7. Adjusts bath blanket to only expose genital area.

8. Removes condom catheter if one if in place.

9. Assists as necessary with perineal care.

10. Attaches collection bag to leg.

11. Moves pubic hair away from penis. Places condom on penis and rolls towards base of penis, leaving space between drainage tip and glans of penis to prevent irritation.

12. Secure condom to penis.

13. Connects catheter tip to drainage tubing. Makes sure tubing is not twisted or kinked.

14. Discards used supplies in plastic bag.

15. Removes and discards gloves.

❏ 16. Washes hands.

❏ 17. Returns bed to its lowest position. Removes bath blanket and store it. Makes client comfortable.

❏ 18. Documents procedure and any observations.

Comments:

Applying warm compresses

✓ **Procedure Steps**

❏ 1. Washes hands.

❏ 2. Explains procedure to client, speaking clearly, slowly, and directly. Maintains face-to-face contact whenever possible.

❏ 3. Provides privacy.

❏ 4. Fills basin with hot water (105° to 110°F). Has client check water temperature and adjust if necessary.

❏ 5. Soaks wash cloth, wrings it out, and applies to area needing compress. Covers with plastic wrap and towel.

❏ 6. Notes the time. Checks area every five minutes. Changes compress if cooling occurs.

❏ 7. Removes compress after 20 minutes, or if area is red, numb, or client complains of pain or discomfort.

❏ 8. Discards water. Cleans and stores basin and other supplies properly. Puts laundry in hamper, and discards plastic wrap.

❏ 9. Washes hands.

❏ 10. Documents time, length, and site of procedure, and any observations.

Comments:

Administering warm soaks

✓ **Procedure Steps**

❏ 1. Washes hands.

❏ 2. Explains procedure to client, speaking clearly, slowly, and directly. Maintains face-to-face contact whenever possible.

❏ 3. Provides privacy.

❏ 4. Fill the basin or tub half full of warm water (105° to 110°F). Has client check water temperature and adjust if necessary.

❏ 5. Immerses body part in water properly, padding the edge of the basin as necessary. Covers client for extra warmth if needed.

❏ 6. Checks water temperature every five minutes, adding hot water as needed.

❏ 7. Observes area for redness and discontinues soak if client complains of pain or discomfort.

❏ 8. Soaks for 15 to 20 minutes or as ordered in the care plan.

❏ 9. Removes basin or helps client out of the tub. Dries the client.

❏ 10. Drains tub or discards water in basin. Cleans and stores basin and other supplies. Puts laundry in hamper.

❏ 11. Washes hands.

❏ 12. Documents time, length, and site of procedure, and any observations. Reports client's response and observations about skin.

Comments:

Using a hot water bottle

✓ **Procedure Steps**

❏ 1. Washes hands.

2. Explains procedure to client, speaking clearly, slowly, and directly. Maintains face-to-face contact whenever possible.

3. Provides privacy.

4. Fills bottle halfway with warm water (105° to 110°F), presses out excess air, and seals bottle.

5. Dries the bottle and checks for leaks. Covers bottle with cloth or towel.

6. Applies bottle to the area. Checks skin every five minutes for redness or pain. Adds cold water to bottle if skin is red or client complains of pain.

7. Removes bottle after 20 minutes or as ordered in the care plan.

8. Empties bottle, and washes and stores supplies.

9. Washes hands.

10. Documents time, length, and site of procedure, and any observations.

Comments:

Assisting with a sitz bath

✓ **Procedure Steps**

1. Washes hands.

2. Explains procedure to client, speaking clearly, slowly, and directly. Maintains face-to-face contact whenever possible.

3. Provides privacy.

4. Puts on gloves.

5. Fills sitz bath two-thirds full with hot water (100°F-104°F or 105°F-110°F, depending on the reason for the bath).

6. Places sitz bath on toilet seat and helps client undress and sit down on sitz bath.

7. Leaves the room and checks on client every five minutes for weakness or dizziness. Stays with client who is unsteady.

8. Assists client out of sitz bath after 20 minutes. Provides towels and helps with dressing as needed.

9. Cleans and stores supplies properly.

10. Removes and discards gloves.

11. Washes hands.

12. Documents procedure, including the time started and ended, the client's response, and the water temperature

Comments:

Applying ice packs

✓ **Procedure Steps**

1. Washes hands.

2. Explains procedure to client, speaking clearly, slowly, and directly. Maintains face-to-face contact whenever possible.

3. Provides privacy.

4. Fills plastic bag with ice and removes excess air. Covers bag with towel.

5. Applies bag to the area as ordered. Uses another towel to cover bag if it is too cold.

6. Notes the time and checks the area after 10 minutes for blisters, pale, white, or gray skin. Stops treatment if client complains of numbness or pain.

7. Removes ice after 20 minutes or as ordered in the care plan. Returns ice bag to freezer.

8. Washes hands.

9. Document the time, length, and site of procedure. Report the client's response and any of your observations about the skin.

Comments:

Applying cold compresses

✓ **Procedure Steps**

☐ 1. Washes hands.

☐ 2. Explains procedure to client, speaking clearly, slowly, and directly. Maintains face-to-face contact whenever possible.

☐ 3. Provides privacy.

☐ 4. Positions client, rinses washcloth in basin, and wrings out washcloth.

☐ 5. Covers the area with sheet or towel and applies cold washcloth to the area. Changes washcloths to keep area cold.

☐ 6. Checks the area after five minutes for blisters, pale, white, or gray skin. Stops treatment if client complains of numbness or pain.

☐ 7. Removes compresses after 20 minutes or as ordered in the care plan. Gives client towels as needed to dry the area.

☐ 8. Cleans and stores basin properly.

☐ 9. Washes hands.

☐ 10. Documents the time, length, and site of procedure. Reports the client's response and any observations about the skin.

Comments:

Changing a dry dressing using non-sterile technique

✓ **Procedure Steps**

☐ 1. Washes hands.

☐ 2. Explains procedure to client, speaking clearly, slowly, and directly. Maintains face-to-face contact whenever possible.

☐ 3. Provides privacy.

☐ 4. Cuts pieces of tape long enough to secure the dressing. Opens gauze package without touching the gauze.

☐ 5. Puts on gloves.

☐ 6. Removes soiled dressing gently, observing dressing for odor or drainage. Notes color of the wound. Disposes of used dressing in the waste bag. Removes and discards gloves in the waste bag.

☐ 7. Puts on new gloves.

☐ 8. Applies clean gauze to wound. Tapes gauze in place.

☐ 9. Removes and discards gloves in the waste bag.

☐ 10. Washes hands.

☐ 11. Documents procedure and any observations.

Comments:

Putting elastic stockings on client

✓ **Procedure Steps**

☐ 1. Washes hands.

☐ 2. Explains procedure to client, speaking clearly, slowly, and directly. Maintains face-to-face contact whenever possible.

☐ 3. Provides privacy.

☐ 4. With client lying down, removes his or her socks, shoes, or slippers, and exposes one leg.

☐ 5. Turns stocking inside-out at least to heel area.

☐ 6. Gently places the foot of the stocking over toes, foot, and heel.

☐ 7. Gently pulls top of stocking over foot, heel, and leg.

☐ 8. Makes sure that there are no twists and wrinkles in the stocking after it is applied.

☐ 9. Repeats for the other leg.

☐ 10. Washes hands.

☐ 11. Documents procedure and any observations.

Comments:

Caring for an ostomy

✓ Procedure Steps

☐ 1. Washes hands.

☐ 2. Explains procedure to client, speaking clearly, slowly, and directly. Maintains face-to-face contact whenever possible.

☐ 3. Provides privacy.

☐ 4. Adjusts the bed to a safe working level, if possible. Locks bed wheels.

☐ 5. Places bed protector under client. Covers client with a bath blanket and only exposes the ostomy site.

☐ 6. Puts on gloves.

☐ 7. Removes ostomy bag carefully. Notes color, odor, consistency, and amount of stool in the bag.

☐ 8. Wipes area around the stoma with toilet paper. Discards paper in plastic bag.

☐ 9. Washes area around the stoma using a washcloth and warm soapy water. Moves in one direction, away from the stoma. Pats dry with another towel. Applies cream if ordered.

☐ 10. Places the clean ostomy appliance on client, following instructions. Makes sure the bottom of the bag is clamped.

☐ 11. Removes disposable bed protector and discards.

☐ 12. Removes and discards gloves. Makes the client comfortable. Puts on fresh gloves and changes linens if necessary. Covers client and removes bath blanket and towel.

☐ 13. Takes bedpan and supplies to bathroom. Empties bag and cleans bag. Cleans bedpan. Stores bedpan and supplies.

☐ 14. Removes and discards gloves.

☐ 15. Washes hands.

☐ 16. Returns bed to lowest position.

☐ 17. Documents procedure and any observations.

Comments:

15

Rehabilitation and Restorative Care

Assisting with passive range of motion exercises

✓ Procedure Steps

☐ 1. Washes hands.

☐ 2. Explains procedure to client, speaking clearly, slowly, and directly. Maintains face-to-face contact whenever possible.

☐ 3. Provides privacy.

☐ 4. Adjusts the bed to a safe working level, if possible. Locks bed wheels.

☐ 5. Positions client in supine position. Repeats each exercise at least three times.

Shoulder:

Performs the following movements properly, supporting the client's arm at the elbow and wrist by placing one hand under the elbow and the other hand under the wrist:

- ❏ 1. Flexion
- ❏ 2. Extension
- ❏ 3. Abduction
- ❏ 4. Adduction

Elbow:

Performs the following movements properly, holding the wrist with one hand, and holding the elbow with the other:

- ❏ 1. Flexion
- ❏ 2. Extension
- ❏ 3. Pronation
- ❏ 4. Supination

Wrist:

Performs the following movements properly, holding the wrist with one hand, and using the fingers of the other hand to help the joint through the motions:

- ❏ 1. Flexion
- ❏ 2. Extension
- ❏ 3. Radial flexion
- ❏ 4. Ulnar flexion

Thumb:

Performs the following movements properly:

- ❏ 1. Abduction
- ❏ 2. Adduction
- ❏ 3. Opposition
- ❏ 4. Flexion
- ❏ 5. Extension

Fingers:

Performs the following movements properly:

- ❏ 1. Flexion
- ❏ 2. Extension
- ❏ 3. Abduction
- ❏ 4. Adduction

Hip:

Performs the following movements properly, placing one hand under the knee and one under the ankle:

- ❏ 1. Abduction
- ❏ 2. Adduction
- ❏ 3. Internal rotation
- ❏ 4. External rotation

Knees:

Performs the following movements properly, placing one hand under the knee and one under the ankle:

- ❏ 1. Flexion
- ❏ 2. Extension

Ankles:

Performs the following movements properly supporting the foot and ankle:

- ❏ 1. Dorsiflexion
- ❏ 2. Plantar flexion
- ❏ 3. Supination
- ❏ 4. Pronation

Toes:

Performs the following movements properly:

- ❏ 1. Flexion
- ❏ 2. Extension
- ❏ 3. Abduction

When all exercises are completed:

- ❏ 6. Returns client to comfortable position and covers as appropriate. Returns bed to lowest position.
- ❏ 7. Washes hands.
- ❏ 8. Documents procedure. Notes any decrease in range of motion or any pain experienced by the client. Notifies supervisor if increased stiffness or physical resistance is noted.

Comments:

16

Medications and Technology in Home Care

Assisting in changing clothes for a client who has an IV

✓ **Procedure Steps**

❑ 1. Washes hands.

❑ 2. Explains procedure to client, speaking clearly, slowly, and directly. Maintains face-to-face contact whenever possible.

❑ 3. Provides privacy.

❑ 4. Adjusts bed to lowest position, if possible, and locks bed wheels. Helps client to sitting position with feet flat on the floor.

❑ 5. Helps client remove the arm without the IV from the clothing.

❑ 6. Helps client gather clothing on arm with IV site, lift clothing over IV site, and move it up the tubing towards the IV bag.

❑ 7. Lifts IV bag off the pole, keeping it higher than the IV site, slides clothing over IV bag, and replaces IV bag on the pole.

❑ 8. Sets used clothing aside and gathers the sleeve of the clean clothing.

❑ 9. Lifts IV bag off the pole again, keeping it higher than the IV site, slides clean clothing over IV bag onto the client's arm, and replaces IV bag on the pole.

❑ 10. Moves clean clothing over tubing and IV site and onto the client's arm.

❑ 11. Assists client with putting other arm into clothing.

❑ 12. Checks the IV, the tubing, and dressing for proper placement.

❑ 13. Assists client with changing the rest of the clothing.

❑ 14. Places soiled laundry in laundry basket, and adjusts bed, if necessary.

Assisting with deep breathing exercises

✓ **Procedure Steps**

❑ 1. Washes hands.

❑ 2. Explains procedure to client, speaking clearly, slowly, and directly. Maintains face-to-face contact whenever possible.

❑ 3. Provides privacy.

❑ 4. Puts on gown, mask, and goggles.

❑ 5. Puts on gloves.

❑ 6. Has client inhale deeply while sitting up.

❑ 7. Has client exhale completely.

❑ 8. Repeats exercise five to ten times.

❑ 9. Offers tissues if necessary.

❑ 10. Disposes of tissues and cleans basin.

❑ 11. Removes gloves, goggles, gown, and mask properly.

❑ 12. Washes hands.

❑ 13. Puts on new gloves.

❑ 14. Provides mouth care.

❑ 15. Removes and discards gloves. Washes hands again.

❑ 16. Documents procedure and any observations.

Comments:

❏ 15. Washes hands.

❏ 16. Documents procedure and any
observations.

Comments:

19

New Mothers, Infants, and Children

Picking up and holding a baby

✓ **Procedure Steps**

❏ 1. Washes hands.

❏ 2. Supports the head at all times when lifting or holding a baby. With the other hand, supports the baby's back and bottom.

❏ 3. Performs cradle hold properly.

❏ 4. Performs football hold properly.

❏ 5. Performs upright hold properly.

Comments:

Sterilizing bottles

✓ **Procedure Steps**

❏ 1. Washes hands.

❏ 2. Boils water and puts equipment in.

❏ 3. Re-boils water for five minutes.

❏ 4. Removes equipment and discards water. Stores when dry.

Comments:

Assisting with bottle feeding

✓ **Procedure Steps**

❏ 1. Washes hands.

❏ 2. Prepares bottle.

❏ 3. Sits and holds baby properly.

❏ 4. Inserts bottle nipple, and ensures that baby's head is higher than body.

❏ 5. Talks or sings to baby during feeding.

❏ 6. Burps baby, changes diaper, and puts baby down.

❏ 7. Washes hands.

❏ 8. Documents procedure and any observations.

❏ 9. Washes and sterilizes bottle.

Comments:

Burping a baby

✓ **Procedure Steps**

❏ 1. Washes hands.

❏ 2. Assembles correct equipment.

❏ 3. Picks baby up, using either of the two safe positions.

❏ 4. Pats back gently until baby burps.

❏ 5. Returns baby to safe position.

Comments:

Giving an infant sponge bath

✓ **Procedure Steps**

❏ 1. Washes hands.

❏ 2. Puts on gloves.

❏ 3. Fills basin and tests temperature.

❏ 4. Holds baby in football hold and washes eyes, then rest of face, using no soap.

❏ 5. Holds baby in football hold and washes hair.

❏ 6. Lays baby down, keeping one hand on baby.

❏ 7. Undresses upper body and washes it. Dries and covers the baby.

❏ 8. Undresses lower body, washes and dries it.

❏ 9. Washes perineal area properly.

❏ 10. Washes bottom and dries completely.

❏ 11. Applies lotion, keeping baby covered.

❏ 12. Diapers and dresses baby. Returns baby to safe position.

❏ 13. Discards water, cleans supplies, and discards gloves.

❏ 14. Washes hands.

❏ 15. Documents procedure and any observations.

Comments:

Giving an infant tub bath

✓ **Procedure Steps**

❏ 1. Washes hands.

❏ 2. Puts on gloves.

❏ 3. Fills basin and tests temperature.

❏ 4. Holds baby in football hold and washes eyes, then rest of face, using no soap.

❏ 5. Holds baby in football hold and washes hair.

❏ 6. Lays baby down, undresses, and immerses baby in basin, keeping head above water.

❏ 7. Uses washcloth to wash from neck down.

❏ 8. Removes from bath and covers immediately.

❏ 9. Applies lotion, keeping baby covered.

❏ 10. Diapers and dresses baby. Returns baby to safe position.

❏ 11. Washes hands.

❏ 12. Documents procedure and any observations.

Comments:

Changing cloth or disposable diapers

✓ **Procedure Steps**

❏ 1. Washes hands.

❏ 2. Puts on gloves.

❏ 3. Undresses baby as necessary and removes diaper.

❏ 4. Cleans perineal area.

❏ 5. Applies ointment as necessary and allows air to circulate.

❏ 6. Applies cloth or disposable diaper properly.

❏ 7. Dresses baby and returns to safe position.

❏ 8. Disposes of diaper properly.

❏ 9. Removes gloves properly.

❏ 10. Washes hands.

❏ 11. Cleans area and stores supplies.

❏ 12. Documents procedure and any observations.

Comments:

Taking an infant's axillary or tympanic temperature

✓ **Procedure Steps**

❑ 1. Washes hands.

❑ 2. Prepares thermometer.

For axillary temperature:

❑ 3. Undresses baby on one side and lays baby down.

❑ 4. Takes temperature, keeping thermometer in place for three to five minutes or until signal sounds.

For tympanic temperature:

❑ 3. Lays baby on side.

❑ 4. Takes temperature, making sure ear is sealed.

❑ 5. Reads temperature, dresses baby, and returns to safe position.

❑ 6. Washes hands.

❑ 7. Documents temperature.

Comments:

20

Common Chronic and Acute Conditions

Providing foot care for the diabetic client

✓ **Procedure Steps**

❑ 1. Washes hands.

❑ 2. Explains procedure to client, speaking clearly, slowly, and directly. Maintains face-to-face contact whenever possible.

❑ 3. Provides privacy.

❑ 4. Puts on gloves.

❑ 5. Washes feet with washcloth and soap, and rinses in warm water.

❑ 6. Pats the feet dry, wiping between the toes.

❑ 7. Gently rubs lotion into the feet with circular strokes.

❑ 8. Observes the skin for signs of dryness, irritation, etc.

❑ 9. Assists client with putting on socks and shoes or slippers.

❑ 10. Disposes of used linens properly and cleans and stores basin and supplies.

❑ 11. Removes and discards gloves.

❑ 12. Washes hands.

❑ 13. Documents procedure and any observations.

Comments:

21

Clean, Safe, and Healthy Environments

Cleaning a bathroom

✓ **Procedure Steps**

❑ 1. Puts on gloves.

❑ 2. Wipes all surfaces with disinfectant and sponge.

❑ 3. Wipes toilet bowl, using different sponge.

❑ 4. Cleans bathtub, shower, and sink, using a different sponge.

❑ 5. Scrubs inside of toilet bowl with brush.

❏ 6. Washes floor.

❏ 7. Cleans mirror and all glass.

❏ 8. Disposes of soiled towels and waste.

❏ 9. Stores supplies. Removes and discards gloves.

❏ 10. Washes hands.

❏ 11. Documents procedure and any observations.

Comments:

Doing the laundry

✓ **Procedure Steps**

❏ 1. Sorts clothes carefully, checking pockets and garments.

❏ 2. Pretreats clothes as necessary.

❏ 3. Uses correct temperature, laundry products, and washing cycle.

❏ 4. Dries clothes.

❏ 5. Hand-washes as necessary.

❏ 6. Folds and hangs clean laundry. Stores clothes.

Comments:

Making an occupied bed

✓ **Procedure Steps**

❏ 1. Washes hands.

❏ 2. Explains procedure to client, speaking clearly, slowly, and directly. Maintains face-to-face contact whenever possible.

❏ 3. Provides privacy.

❏ 4. Places clean linen within reach.

❏ 5. Adjusts the bed to a safe working level, if possible. Locks bed wheels.

❏ 6. Puts on gloves.

❏ 7. Covers client and loosens top linen from working side. Removes top sheet.

❏ 8. Raises side rail on far side of bed and rolls client onto her side.

❏ 9. Loosens bottom soiled linen, mattress pad, and protector on working side.

❏ 10. Rolls bottom soiled linen toward client, tucking it snugly against the client's back.

❏ 11. Places and tucks in clean bottom linen, finishing with no wrinkles. Makes hospital corners if necessary.

❏ 12. Smoothes bottom sheet out toward the client. Rolls extra material toward client and tucks it under client's body.

❏ 13. Places waterproof pad if using and centers it. Smoothes it out toward client, and tucks it under client's body.

❏ 14. Places draw sheet if using. Smoothes and tucks as with other bedding.

❏ 15. Raises side rail nearest self and lowers side rail on other side of bed. Assists client to turn onto clean bottom sheet.

❏ 16. Loosens soiled linen. Rolls linen from head to the foot of bed, avoiding contact with skin or clothes. Places it in a laundry hamper or basket.

❏ 17. Pulls and tucks in clean bottom linen just like other side, finishing with bottom sheet free of wrinkles.

❏ 18. Asks client to turn onto his or her back, keeping client covered. Raises side rail.

❏ 19. Unfolds top sheet and places it over client. Slips blanket or old sheet out from underneath. Puts it in the laundry hamper.

❏ 20. Places a blanket over the top sheet, matching the top edges. Tucks bottom edges of top sheet and blanket under mattress, making square corners on each side. Loosens top linens over client's feet. Folds top sheet over the blanket about six inches.

❏ 21. Removes pillow and pillowcase. Places it in the laundry hamper. Removes gloves.

❏ 22. Places clean pillowcases on pillows. Places them under client's head.

❏ 23. Returns bed to lowest position. Carries laundry hamper to laundry area.

❏ 24. Washes hands.

❏ 25. Documents procedure and any observations.

Comments:

Making an unoccupied bed

✓ Procedure Steps

❏ 1. Washes hands.

❏ 2. Places clean linen within reach.

❏ 3. Adjusts the bed to a safe working level, if possible. Locks bed wheels.

❏ 4. Puts on gloves.

❏ 5. Loosens soiled linen and rolls it from head to foot of bed. Avoids contact with skin or clothes. Places it in a hamper or basket.

❏ 6. Removes and discards gloves. Washes hands.

❏ 7. Remakes bed, spreading mattress pad and bottom sheet, tucking under. Makes hospital corners. Puts on mattress protector and draw sheet, smoothes, and tucks under sides of bed.

❏ 8. Places top sheet and blanket, centering them. Tucks under end of bed and makes hospital corners. Folds down top sheet over the blanket about six inches.

❏ 9. Removes pillows and pillowcases. Puts on clean pillowcases. Replaces pillows.

❏ 10. Returns bed to its lowest position. Carries laundry hamper to laundry area.

❏ 11. Washes hands.

❏ 12. Documents procedure and any observations.

Comments:

23

Meal Planning, Shopping, Preparation, and Storage

Assisting a client with eating

✓ Procedure Steps

❏ 1. Washes hands.

❏ 2. Explains procedure to client, speaking clearly, slowly, and directly. Maintains face-to-face contact whenever possible.

❏ 3. Assist client to wash hands.

❏ 4. Adjust bed height to sit at client's eye level. Locks bed wheels.

❏ 5. Ensures client is in upright sitting position. Assists client to put on clothing protector, if desired.

❏ 6. Sits at client's eye level on stronger side.

❏ 7. Checks temperature of food. Offers food in bite-sized pieces and alternates types of food offered. Makes sure client's mouth is empty before offering the next bite of food or sip of drink.

❏ 8. Offers drinks throughout the meal. Talks throughout the meal.

❏ 9. Wipes client's mouth and hands as necessary.

❏ 10. Removes clothing protector if used. Removes tray or dishes.

❏ 11. Assists client to a comfortable position. Return bed to lowest position.

❏ 12. Washes hands.

❏ 13. Documents procedure (including client's intake, if required) and any observations.

Comments:

Notes

Notes

Notes

Notes